CliffsTestPrep®

ELM & EPT

CliffsTestPrep®

ELM & EPT

by

Jerry Bobrow, Ph.D.

Contributing Authors

Jean Eggensehwiler, M.A.

George Crowder, M.A.

Dale Johnson, M.A.

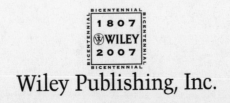

Wiley Publishing, Inc.

About the Author

Jerry Bobrow, Ph.D., is a national authority in the field of test preparation. As executive director of Bobrow Test Preparation Services, he has been administering test preparation programs at more than 25 California institutions for the past 31 years. Dr. Bobrow has authored more than 40 national best-selling test preparation books, and his books and programs have assisted more than two million test-takers.

Publisher's Acknowledgments

Editorial

Project Editor: Donna Wright

Acquisitions Editor: Greg Tubach

Production

Proofreader: Henry Lazarek

Wiley Publishing, Inc. Composition Services

CliffsTestPrep® ELM & EPT

Published by:
Wiley Publishing, Inc.
111 River Street
Hoboken, NJ 07030-5774
www.wiley.com

Copyright © 2007 Jerry Bobrow, Ph.D.

Published by Wiley, Hoboken, NJ
Published simultaneously in Canada

Library of Congress Cataloging-in-Publication Data

Bobrow, Jerry.

CliffsTestPrep ELM & EPT / by Jerry Bobrow.

   p. cm.

 ISBN-13: 978-0-471-78678-8

 ISBN-10: 0-471-78678-0

 1. Universities and colleges—California—Entrance examinations—Study guides. 2. California State University—Entrance examinations—Study guides. 3. Mathematics—Examinations—Study guides. 4. English language—Examinations—Study guides. I. Title. II. Title: CliffsTestPrep ELM and EPT.

 LB2353.24.C2B63 2007

 378.1'662--dc22

                  2006027032

Printed in the United States of America

10 9 8 7 6 5 4 3 2 1

1O/TR/RQ/QW/IN

WILEY

Table of Contents

PART III: TWO SIMULATED ELM PRACTICE TESTS

PART IV: ANALYSIS OF THE EPT EXAM AREAS

PART V: SIMULATED EPT PRACTICE TEST

PART VI: FINAL PREPARATION

Preface

We know that doing well on the ELM and EPT are important to you!

And we can help.

As a matter of fact, we have spent the last 30 years helping over a million test-takers successfully prepare for important exams. The techniques and strategies that students and adults have found most effective in our preparation programs at 26 universities, county offices of education, and school districts make this book your key to success on the ELM and EPT.

Our easy-to-use ELM and EPT Preparation Guide gives you that *extra edge* by:

- ❑ Answering commonly asked questions
- ❑ Introducing important test-taking strategies and techniques
- ❑ Including diagnostic tests in arithmetic, algebra, and geometry to help you pinpoint your weaknesses
- ❑ Reviewing the basics skills necessary in arithmetic, algebra, and geometry
- ❑ Analyzing sample problems and giving suggested approaches on the ELM and EPT
- ❑ Reviewing the writing process
- ❑ Providing three simulated practice exams (2 ELM and 1 EPT) with explanations
- ❑ Including analysis charts to help you spot your strengths and weaknesses.

We give you lots of strategies and techniques with plenty of practice problems.

There is no substitute for working hard in your regular classes, doing all of your homework and assignments, and preparing properly for your classroom exams and finals. But if you want that *extra edge* to do your best on the ELM and EPT, then this guide can be your key to success.

Best of Luck,
Jerry Bobrow, Ph.D.

Introduction

Format of the ELM

The test consists of 50 multiple-choice questions; 45 of the questions actually count toward your score. The following areas are covered (but the questions will **not be labeled or in this order**):

Format of the Entry Level Mathematics (ELM)	
Number Sense and Data	15–20 Questions
Algebra	15–20 Questions
Geometry	13–17 Questions
Total	50 Questions

Total time for the ELM is 90 minutes or 1 hour and 30 minutes.

The number of questions and the types of questions may be adjusted slightly in later tests. Also note that the five "trial" questions could be scattered anywhere on the exam.

The test is scored from 0–80 with a passing scaled score of 50.

Subscores are given for Number Sense and Data, Algebra, and Geometry.

Format of the EPT

The test consists of one essay (45 minutes), a reading skills section (30 minutes), and a composing skills section (30 minutes). The following areas are covered:

Format of the English Placement Test (EPT)		
Essay	1 Essay Question	45 Minutes
Reading Skills	45 Multiple-Choice Questions	30 Minutes
Composing Skills	45 Multiple-Choice Questions	30 Minutes
Total	1 Essay Question and 90 Multiple-Choice Questions	

Total time for the EPT is 105 minutes or 1 hour and 45 minutes.

The number of questions and the types of questions may be adjusted slightly in later tests. Also note that "trial" questions could be scattered anywhere on the exam.

The essay is scored from 2 (low) to 12 (high). The reading skills and composing skills are each scored from 120–180. The total score of the test is scaled to 120–180.

How You Can Do Your Best

A Positive Approach

Since every question is worth the same number of points, do the easy ones first. To do your best, use this positive approach:

1. First, look for the questions that you can answer and should get right.
2. Next, skip the ones that give you a lot of trouble. (But take a guess.)
3. Remember, don't get stuck on any one of the questions.

Here's a closer look at this system:

1. Answer the easy questions as soon as you see them.
2. When you come to a question that gives you trouble, don't get stuck.
3. Before you go to the next question, try to eliminate some of the incorrect choices to that question. Then take a guess from the choices left!
4. If you can't eliminate some choices, take a guess anyway. Never leave a question unanswered.
5. Put a check mark in your test booklet next to the number of a problem for which you did not know the answer and simply guessed.
6. After you answer all the questions, go back to work on the ones that you checked (the ones that you guessed on the first time through).

Don't ever leave a question without taking a guess. There is no penalty for guessing.

The Elimination Strategy

Sometimes the best way to get the right answer is by eliminating the wrong answers. As you read your answer choices, keep the following in mind:

1. Eliminate wrong answer choices right away.
2. Mark them out in your question booklet.
3. If you feel that you know the right answer when you spot it, mark it. You don't need to look at all the rest of the choices (although a good strategy for some questions is to scan the choices first).
4. Try to narrow your choices down to two so that you can take a better guess.

Remember, getting rid of the wrong choices can leave you with the right choice. Look for the right answer choice and eliminate wrong answer choices.

Here's a closer look at the elimination strategy.

Take advantage of being allowed to mark in your testing booklet. As you eliminate an answer choice from consideration, make sure to mark it out in your question booklet as follows:

A̶

?B

C̶

?D

E̶

Notice that some choices are marked with question marks, signifying that they may be possible answers. This technique will help you avoid reconsidering those marked-out choices you have already eliminated and will help you narrow down your possible answers. These marks in your testing booklet **do not need to be erased**.

Avoiding the Misread

One of the most common errors is the misread, that is, when you simply misread the question.

For example,

An ELM question could ask,

If $6x + 3y = 14$, what is the value of y?

The question may instead have asked, "What is the value of x?"

or

If $3x + x = 20$, what is the value of $x + 2$?

Notice that this question doesn't ask for the value of x, but rather the value of $x + 2$.

An EPT question could ask,

What does the word "lifting" mean in the context of the passage?

Notice that this question asks for the meaning of "lifting" in the context of the passage.

or

Which of the following is the main point of the passage?

Notice that here you are looking for the *main* point.

To avoid misreading a question (and therefore answering it incorrectly), simply circle or underline what you must answer in the question. For example, do you have to find x or $x + 2$? Do you have to know the meaning of the word "lifting" or can you find its meaning in the passage? To help you avoid misreads, circle or underline the questions in your test booklet in this way:

If $6x + 3y = 14$, what is the <u>value of y</u>?

If $3x + x = 20$, what is the <u>value of $x + 2$</u>?

What does the word "<u>lifting</u>" mean in the <u>context of the passage</u>?

Which of the following is the <u>main point</u> of the passage?

And, once again, these circles or underlines in your question booklet do not have to be erased.

A Quick Review of Basic Strategies

1. Do the easy problems first.
2. Don't get stuck on one problem—they're all of equal value.
3. On elimination answers—mark out wrong answer choices in your test booklet.
4. Avoid misreading a question—circle or underline important words.
5. Take advantage of being allowed to write in the test booklet.
6. No penalty for guessing means "never leave a question without at least taking a guess."

Questions Commonly Asked About the ELM and EPT

Q. Is the ELM or the EPT an admission test?

A. No. The ELM and EPT are placement tests. They are designed to measure skill levels of entering California State University students in math and English.

Q. Who must take the ELM and/or EPT?

A. All undergraduate students admitted to a California State University are required to take the ELM and/or EPT unless they qualify for exemption. Check with your California State University (CSU) Admissions Office to see if you qualify for one of the exemptions.

Q. When should I take the ELM and/or EPT?

A. Take the ELM and/or EPT as soon as possible after admission, unless your school requests an earlier test. You must take the test before you enroll.

Q. How do I register?

A. If you have not received a copy of the registration form in the mail, you may pick one up at any CSU Admissions Office. The registration form must be mailed to the test office on the campus where you wish to attend. Be sure to contact the campus where you plan to take the test because campuses have different registration requirements. At some campuses you can register online.

Q. Where will the ELM and EPT be given?

A. The ELM and EPT will be given at all CSU campuses. You may register to take the test at whichever campus you choose; it does not have to be the campus you plan to attend.

Q. When are the ELM and EPT given?

A. All 23 CSU campuses administer the tests on the statewide dates (three times). Many campuses have additional test dates. This information is available at www.ets.org and click "Tests directory."

Q. How long should I plan on being at the testing center?

A. Plan on a minimum of 2 hours for the ELM (90 minutes of testing time) and 2½ hours for the EPT (105 minutes of testing time).

Q. What is a passing score?

A. As mentioned earlier, the ELM and the EPT are placement tests. They use "cut scores" to place you in appropriate mathematics and English classes. If you score at or above the cut score of 50 on the ELM, which is scored from 0–80, then you will be placed in regular, college-level math classes. If you score below 50, you will need to take remedial coursework in math. The subscores given for Number Sense and Data, Algebra, and Geometry will provide guidance in determining your remediation coursework.

The cut score for the EPT is 151 on a scale that goes from 120 to 180 (lowest-highest). If you score at or above the cut score, you will be placed in regular, college-level English classes. If you score below 151, you will need to take remedial coursework in English. Scores for the component parts of the EPT are also given—Reading Skills (120–180), Composing Skills (120–180), and the Essay (1–6).

Q. When will I get my scores?

A. An individual student score report will be mailed to you at the address you provide on the day of the test.

Q. What must I take to the test center?

A. You must bring your validated admission ticket, your social security number, acceptable identification, a check or money order payable to ETS for test fees, several No. 2 lead pencils with erasers, two ballpoint pens for writing the EPT essay. (You may bring a silent watch and a bag or backpack, if you wish.)

Q. What can't I take with me to the test center?

A. You may NOT take books, calculators, rulers, papers of any kind, personal digital assistants (PDA), cellular telephones, pagers, or any photographic devices. Eating, drinking, and smoking are NOT permitted in the buildings.

Q. May I use a calculator during the ELM exam?

A. No. The questions do not require long computations, so a calculator is not necessary.

Q. Do I get scratch paper for working the problems?

A. No. All of your work will be done in the testing booklet, but you must transfer your answer as you complete each question onto a special answer sheet.

Q. How should I prepare?

A. Keep up with class work and homework in your regular classes. There is no substitute for a sound education. If you have not taken a math or English class recently, start your review early, a few months before the tests. If you are presently taking math and English classes, you can start a little closer to your test date. In either case, using an organized test preparation approach is very important. Carefully follow the Study Plan in this book for the ELM and EPT to give you that organized approach. It will show you how to apply techniques and strategies and help focus your review. Carefully reviewing sample exam problems available free online will also give you an edge in doing your best.

Q. Should I guess on the tests?

A. Yes! Since there is no penalty for guessing, guess if you have to. If possible, try to eliminate some of the choices to increase your chances of choosing the right answer.

Q. How can I get more information?

A. More information and released exam questions can be found at www.ets.org/csu/elm.html or www.ets.org/csu/ept.html.

PART I

ANALYSIS OF THE ELM EXAM AREAS

Introduction to the Entry Level Mathematics (ELM)

The purpose of the Entry Level Mathematics is to determine whether you are prepared to undertake college-level work in mathematics. The results of the test will be used to place you in the appropriate course.

The ELM is composed of 50 multiple-choice questions; 45 of the questions actually count toward your score. You have 90 minutes to complete the test. The following areas are covered (but the questions will **not be labeled or in this order**):

Contents of the Entry Level Mathematics (ELM)	
Number Sense and Data	35% or about 15–20 Questions
Algebra	35% or about 15–20 Questions
Geometry	30% or about 13–17 Questions
Total	50 Questions

Total time for the ELM is 90 minutes or 1 hour and 30 minutes.

The number of questions and the types of questions may be adjusted slightly in later tests. Also note that the five "trial" questions could be scattered anywhere on the exam.

Scoring the ELM

Remember, the ELM is a placement test. It uses "cut scores" to place you in appropriate mathematics classes. If you score at or above the cut score of 50 on the ELM, which is scored from 0–80, then you will be placed in regular, college-level math classes. If you score below 50, you will need to take remedial coursework in math. The subscores given for Number Sense and Data, Algebra, and Geometry will provide guidance in determining your remediation coursework.

Basic Skills and Concepts You Should Be Familiar With

The following list will give you an indication of the basic skills and topics you should be familiar with to pass the ELM. You may wish to use this official list of ELM Topics as a checklist when you begin your review.

CSU ELM Topics

NUMBER SENSE AND DATA (approximately 35%)

- ❏ Carry out basic arithmetic calculations
- ❏ Understand and use percent in context
- ❏ Compare and order rational numbers expressed as fractions and/or decimals
- ❏ Solve problems involving fractions and/or decimals in context
- ❏ Interpret and use ratio and proportion in context
- ❏ Use estimation appropriately
- ❏ Evaluate the reasonableness of a solution to a problem
- ❏ Evaluate and estimate square roots
- ❏ Represent and understand data presented graphically (including pie charts, bar and line graphs, histograms, and other formats for presenting data visually used in print and electronic media)
- ❏ Calculate and understand the arithmetic mean
- ❏ Calculate and understand the median
- ❏ Make estimates and predictions based on data
- ❏ Distinguish between reasonable and unreasonable claims based on data

ALGEBRA (approximately 35%)

- ❏ Evaluate and interpret algebraic expressions
- ❏ Simplify algebraic expressions
- ❏ Express relationships among quantities using variables
- ❏ Use properties of exponents
- ❏ Perform polynomial arithmetic (add, subtract, multiply, divide, and factor)
- ❏ Perform arithmetic operations involving rational expressions
- ❏ Solve linear equations (with both numerical and literal coefficients)
- ❏ Solve systems of linear equations in two unknowns
- ❏ Solve linear inequalities
- ❏ Solve problems in context that are modeled by linear equations
- ❏ Solve quadratic and rational equations (with both numerical and literal coefficients; real solutions only)
- ❏ Solve problems in context that are modeled by quadratic equations
- ❏ Solve equations involving absolute value (in one variable)
- ❏ Solve inequalities involving absolute value (in one variable)
- ❏ Find and use slopes and intercepts of lines
- ❏ Use constant and average rates to solve problems in context (using appropriate units)

GEOMETRY (approximately 30%)

❏ Find the perimeter, area, or volume of geometric figures (including triangles, quadrilaterals, rectangular parallelepipeds, circles, cylinders, and combinations of these figures)

❏ Calculate the ratio of corresponding geometric measurements of similar figures (e.g., if the perimeters are in a 3:2 ratio, the areas are in a 9:4 ratio)

❏ Use the Pythagorean Theorem

❏ Use properties of congruent or similar geometric objects

❏ Solve geometric problems using the properties of basic geometric figures (including triangles, quadrilaterals, polygons, and circles)

❏ Determine angles in the plane (using properties of intersecting lines, parallel lines, and perpendicular lines)

❏ Identify and plot points on the number line

❏ Identify and plot points in the coordinate plane

❏ Plot points on the graph of a function determined by an algebraic expression

❏ Graph linear functions in one variable

❏ Graph quadratic functions in one variable

❏ Relate basic information about a function to features of its graph (e.g., linearity, positivity or negativity, increasing or decreasing)

❏ Find the length or midpoint of a line segment in the coordinate plane

Strategies and Samples

Carefully review the following strategies and sample problems. They will help give you insight into how to approach many different question types.

Circle or Underline

Take advantage of being allowed to mark on the test booklet by always underlining or circling what you are looking for. This will ensure that you are answering the right question.

Samples

---

1. If $x + 6 = 9$, then $3x + 1 =$

    A.   3
    B.   9
    C. 10
    D. 34
    E. 46

You should first circle or underline $3x + 1$ because this is what you are solving for. Solving for x leaves $x = 3$, then substituting into $3x + 1$ gives $3(3) + 1$, 10. The most common mistake is to solve for x, which is 3, and *mistakenly choose A* as your answer. But remember, you are solving for $3x + 1$, not just x. You should also notice that most of the other choices would all be possible answers if you made common or simple mistakes. *Make sure that you are answering the right question.* The correct answer is C.

---

2. Together, a hat and coat cost $125. The coat costs $25 more than the hat. What is the cost of the coat?

    A. $25
    B. $50
    C. $75
    D. $100
    E. $125

The key words here are cost of the coat, so circle those words. To solve algebraically,

$$x = \text{hat}$$
$$x + \$25 = \text{coat (cost \$25 more than the hat)}$$

Together they cost $125.

$$(x + 25) + x = 125$$
$$2x + 25 = 125$$
$$2x = 100$$
$$x = 50$$

But this is the cost of the hat. Notice that $50 is one of the answer choices, B. Since $x = 50$, then $x + 25 = 75$. Therefore, the coat costs $75, which is Choice C. *Always answer the question that is being asked.* Circling the key word or words will help you do that. The correct answer is C.

3. Which of the following is between $\frac{1}{4}$ and 0.375?

    A. 0.0094

    B. 0.291

    C. 0.38

    D. 0.4

    E. 0.51

First underline the word "between." Next simplify $\frac{1}{4}$ to .25. A quick glance at the choices is valuable because it tips you off that you are working in decimals. Simply check which decimal is between .250 and .375. The correct answer is B—.291 is between .250 and .375. Notice that changing .25 to .250 makes the problem even easier. (Adding or eliminating zeros to the far right of a decimal doesn't change the value of the number.)

Pull Out Information

Pulling information out of the word problem structure can often give you a better look at what you are working with; therefore, you gain additional insight into the problem.

Samples

---

1. Phil works for a furniture store $\frac{3}{4}$ of the year and for a pool supply store for $\frac{1}{6}$ of the same year. He takes a vacation for the remainder of the year. How much more time does he spend working for the furniture store than for the pool supply store?

   A. 1 month
   B. 2 months
   C. 7 months
   D. 9 months
   E. 11 months

First circle or underline "How much more time." Next, pull out the information regarding Phil's work for the year:

furniture store $\frac{3}{4}$ of a year is $\frac{3}{4} \times 12$, or 9 months

pool supply store $\frac{1}{6}$ of a year, or $\frac{2}{12}$, which is 2 months

The difference is 9 months minus 2 months, which is 7 months. The correct answer is C. Notice that taking a quick look at the answer choices is helpful, letting you know that the answer is in months.

---

2. If the ratio of boys to girls in a drama class is 2 to 1, which of the following is a possible number of students in the class?

   A. 10
   B. 16
   C. 19
   D. 25
   E. 30

First underline or circle "possible number of students." Then, pulling out information gives you the following.

$b:g = 2:1$

Because the ratio of boys to girls is 2:1, the possible total number of students in the class must be a multiple of 2 + 1 (boys plus girls), or 3. The multiples of 3 are 3, 6, 9, 12, 15 and so on. Only Choice E, 30, is a multiple of 3.

Work Forward

If you quickly see the method to solve the problem, then do the work. Work forward.

Samples

1. $\dfrac{10^{-3}}{10^{-6}} =$

    A. 10^{-3}
    B. 10^{-2}
    C. 10^{2}
    D. 10^{3}
    E. 10^{4}

This is a straightforward mechanical problem. You must know the rules for dividing numbers of the same base with exponents. When you divide numbers with exponents and the bases of the numbers are the same, then you keep the same base and subtract the exponents. For example, x^a divided by x^b is x^{a-b}.

In this case, $= \dfrac{10^{-3}}{10^{-6}} = 10^{-3} \div 10^{-3}(^{-6}) = 10^{-3+6} = 10^{3}$

The correct answer is D.

2. If $|x| = 6$, what is the value of x?

    A. -6 or 0
    B. -6 or 6
    C. 0 or 6
    D. 0 or 12
    E. 12 or -12

You can work this problem forward, using the definition of absolute value. If you know that absolute value refers to actual distance on a number line, and not direction, then it is evident that x can be -6 or 6. The correct answer is B.

You can also work this problem by plugging in the answers, but you still need to know how to work with absolute values.

3. If $x = 3$ and $y = 5$, then $6x^2 - 4y =$

    A. 16
    B. 34
    C. 54
    D. 60
    E. 64

To evaluate an expression, simply plug in the given numbers or values. These types of problems are usually easy to solve as long as you are careful in your calculations and understand the order of operations. Plugging in the values given for x and y:

$$6x^2 - 4y =$$
$$6(3)^2 - 4(5) =$$
$$6(9) - 4(5) =$$
$$54 - 20 = 34$$

The correct answer is B.

Remember, the order of operations is

> **P**arentheses
>
> **E**xponents
>
> **M**ultiplication or **D**ivision
>
> **A**ddition or **S**ubtraction

A good tool for remembering the order of operations is **PEMDAS.**

Work Backward

In some instances, it will be easier to work from the answers. Do not disregard this method because it will at least eliminate some of the choices and could give you the correct answer.

Samples

1. Which of the following points is the y-intercept of the line $3x + 2y = 6$?

    A. (2, 0)
    B. (2, 1)
    C. (0, 2)
    D. (0, 3)
    E. (3, 0)

Probably the fastest method to answer this question is working from the answers. First, note that you are looking for the y-intercept. The y-intercept is where the line crosses the y-axis, so x must be 0. Eliminate choices A, B, and E because the x coordinate is not 0. Next, plug in choices C and D to see which is true for the equation.

Choice C (0, 2):

$$3x + 2y = 6$$
$$3(0) + 2(2) \; ? \; 6$$
$$0 + 4 \neq 6$$

So you can eliminate C. The correct answer is D.

Choice D (0, 3):

$$3x + 2y = 6$$
$$3(0) + 2(3) \; ? \; 6$$
$$0 + 6 = 6$$

Another method for solving this problem is to change the equation of the line to slope-intercept form, $y = mx + b$, where b is the y-intercept.

$$3x + 2y = 6$$

Subtract $3x$ from each side.

$$\begin{array}{rcr} 3x + 2y & = & 6 \\ -3x & & -3x \\ \hline 2y & = & -3x + 6 \end{array}$$

Divide both sides by 2.

$$\frac{2y}{2} = \frac{-3x}{2} + \frac{6}{2}$$
$$y = \left(\frac{-3}{2}\right)x + 3$$

So the y-intercept is 3.

2. Mr. Tuchman can paint 30 surfboards in an hour. Mr. Christianson can paint 60 surfboards in an hour. If they are both painting surfboards, how long does it take them to paint a total of 45 surfboards?

    A.   30 minutes
    B.   45 minutes
    C.   60 minutes
    D.   90 minutes
    E.   120 minutes

You are looking for *how long it takes to paint 45 surfboards if both men are painting.* You can work this problem from the answers. First, try Choice A, 30 minutes. If Mr. Tuchman can paint 30 surfboards in an hour, then he can paint 15 surfboards in half an hour. If Mr. Christianson can paint 60 surfboards in an hour, then he can paint 30 surfboards in half an hour.

So, together they can paint 45 surfboards in 30 minutes. The correct answer is A.

You can also work this problem algebraically. If t is the number of hours, and Mr. Tuchman paints at a rate of 30 surfboards an hour, this can be expressed as $30t$. If Mr. Christianson paints at a rate of 60 surfboards an hour, then this can be expressed as $60t$. They both have to work to paint a total of 45 surfboards, so you can set up the equation $30t + 60t = 45$. Now, solve as follows:

$$30t + 60t = 45$$
$$90t = 45$$

Dividing by 90 gives
$$t = \frac{45}{90}$$

So, $t = \frac{1}{2}$ hour, or 30 minutes. The correct answer is A.

3. The square root of 90 is between

    A.   9 and 10
    B.   10 and 11
    C.   11 and 12
    D.   12 and 13
    E.   13 and 14

This problem is most easily answered by working backward from the answers. Start with Choice A, 9 and 10. If you square 9, that is, 9×9, you get 81, which is below 90. Next, try squaring the second number, 10, and you get 100. Since 90 is between 81 and 100, the square root of 90 is between 9 and 10. The correct answer is A.

You can work this problem forward by approximating the square root of 90. First, find the closest perfect square number below 90. That is 81. Next, find the closest perfect square number above 90, which is 100.

Since $\sqrt{90}$ is between $\sqrt{81}$ and $\sqrt{100}$, it falls somewhere between 9 and 10.

$$\overset{9}{\sqrt{81}} < \sqrt{90} < \overset{10}{\sqrt{100}}$$

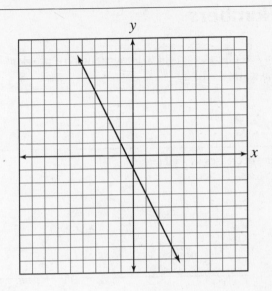

4. Which of the following is the equation of the line shown in the preceding graph?

    A. $y = 2x + 1$
    B. $y = 2x + 2$
    C. $y = -2x - 1$
    D. $y = -2x - 2$
    E. $y = -2x - 3$

A quick look at the choices lets you eliminate some by looking for the y-intercept first. Since the line crosses the y-axis at −1, the y-intercept on the graph is −1. You can eliminate choices A, B, D, and E. The correct answer is C.

In this question, you don't even need to deal with the slopes. But if you are working with the slopes, you can eliminate choices A and B immediately because they are positive. Since the line goes down to the right, the slope is negative.

Substitute Simple Numbers

Substituting numbers for variables can often be an aid to understanding a problem. Remember to substitute simple numbers, since you have to do the work.

Sample

1. If $x > 1$, which of the following decreases as x increases?

    A. $x + x^2$
    B. $2x^2 - x$
    C. $2x - x^2$
    D. $x^3 - 3x$
    E. $x^4 - 4x$

This problem is most easily solved by taking each situation and substituting in simple numbers. However, in the first situation, A, $x + x^2$, you should recognize that this expression will increase as x increases. So you can eliminate A.

Next, Choice B. Trying $x = 2$ in the expression $2x^2 - x$ gives $2(2)^2 - 2$, or $2(4) - 2 = 6$.

Now trying $x = 3$ in the expression gives $2(3)^2 - 3 = 2(9) - 3 = 18 - 3 = 15$.

This expression also increases as x increases. Therefore, eliminate B.

Next, Choice C.

Trying $x = 2$ gives $2(2) - (2)^2 = 4 - 4 = 0$.

Now trying $x = 3$ gives $2(3) - (3)^2 = 6 - 9 = -3$.

So the correct answer is C.

Be sure to make logical substitutions. Use a positive number, a negative number, or zero when applicable to get the full picture.

Be Reasonable

Sometimes you will immediately recognize a simple method to solve a problem. If this is not the case, try a reasonable approach and then check the answers to see which one is most reasonable.

Samples

1. Barney can mow the lawn in 5 hours, and Fred can mow the lawn in 4 hours. How long will it take them to mow the lawn together?

   A. 5 hours

   B. $4\frac{1}{2}$ hours

   C. 4 hours

   D. $2\frac{2}{9}$ hours

   E. 1 hour

Suppose that you are unfamiliar with the type of equation for this problem. Try the "reasonable" method. Since Fred can mow the lawn in 4 hours by himself, it will take less than 4 hours if Barney helps him. Therefore, choices A, B, and C are ridiculous. Taking this method a little further, suppose that Barney could also mow the lawn in 4 hours. Then, together it would take Barney and Fred 2 hours. But since Barney is a little slower than this, the total time should be a little more than 2 hours. The correct answer is D, $2\frac{2}{9}$ hours.

Using the equation for this problem would give the following calculations:

$$\frac{1}{5} + \frac{1}{4} = \frac{1}{x}$$

In 1 hour, Barney could do $\frac{1}{5}$ of the job, and in 1 hour, Fred could do $\frac{1}{4}$ of the job. Unknown $\frac{1}{x}$ is that part of the job they could do together in 1 hour. Now solving, you calculate as follows:

$$\frac{4}{20} + \frac{5}{20} = \frac{1}{x}$$

Cross multiplying gives $\qquad\qquad\qquad 9x = 20$

Therefore, $\qquad\qquad\qquad\qquad x = \frac{20}{9}$ or $2\frac{2}{9}$

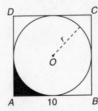

2. Circle O is inscribed in square $ABCD$ as shown above. The area of the shaded region is approximately

   A. 10

   B. 25

   C. 30

   D. 50

   E. 75

Using a reasonable approach, you would first find the area of the square: $10 \times 10 = 100$. Then divide the square into four equal sections as follows:

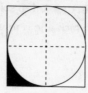

Since a quarter of the square is 25, then the shaded region must be much less than 25. The only possible answer is Choice A, 10.

Another approach to this problem would be to first find the area of the square: $10 \times 10 = 100$. Then subtract the approximate area of the circle:

$$A = \pi(r^2) \cong 3(5^2) = 3(25) = 75.$$

Therefore, the total area inside the square but outside the circle is approximately 25. One quarter of that area is shaded. Therefore, $\frac{25}{4}$ is approximately the shaded area. The closest answer is A, 10.

Sketch a Diagram

Sketching diagrams or simple pictures can also be very helpful in problem solving because the diagram may tip off either a simple solution or a method for solving the problem.

Samples

1. What is the maximum number of milk cartons, each 2" wide by 3" long by 4" tall, that can be fit into a cardboard box with inside dimensions of 16" wide by 9" long by 8" tall?

    A. 12
    B. 18
    C. 20
    D. 24
    E. 48

Drawing a diagram, as shown below, may be helpful in envisioning the process of fitting the cartons into the box. Notice that eight cartons will fit across the box, three cartons deep, and two "stacks" high:

$$8 \times 3 \times 2 = 48 \text{ cartons}$$

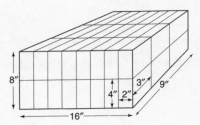

The correct answer is E.

2. If the area of one face of a cube is 16 square inches, what is the volume of the cube in cubic inches?

    A. 8
    B. 12
    C. 24
    D. 64
    E. 96

First underline or circle the word "volume." Now draw a cube.

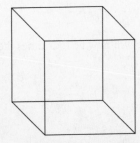

Next, label one face of the cube. This helps you determine that each edge of the cube is 4 inches because the face of a cube is square and all edges are equal.

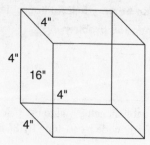

The formula for the volume of a cube is length times width times height, or $V = lwh$.

So the volume is $4 \times 4 \times 4 = 64$, which is Choice D.

Keep in mind that in a cube all edges are the same length and all six sides have the same area.

---

3. If all sides of a square are doubled, the area of that square:

    A. is doubled.
    B. is tripled.
    C. is multiplied by 4.
    D. remains the same.
    E. is multiplied by 8

One way to solve this problem is to draw a square and then double all its sides. Then compare the two areas.

Your first diagram

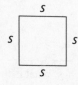

Doubling every side

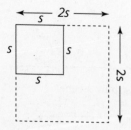

You can see that the total area of the new square will now be four times the original square. The correct answer is C.

Mark in Diagrams

Marking in or labeling diagrams as you read the questions can save you valuable time. Marking can also give you insight into how to solve a problem because you will have the complete picture clearly in front of you.

Samples

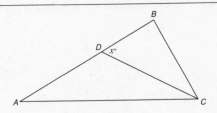

1. In the triangle above, *CD* is an angle bisector, angle *ACD* is 30°, and angle *ABC* is a right angle. What is the measurement of angle *x* in degrees?

   A.   30°
   B.   45°
   C.   60°
   D.   75°
   E.   80°

You should have read the problem and marked as follows: In the triangle above, *CD* is an angle bisector (*stop and mark in the drawing*), angle *ACD* is 30° (*stop and mark in the drawing*), and angle *ABC* is a right angle (*stop and mark in the drawing*). What is the measurement of angle *x* in degrees? (*Stop and mark in or circle what you are looking for in the drawing.*)

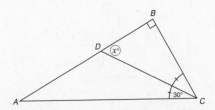

Now, with the drawing marked in, it is evident that, since angle *ACD* is 30°, then angle *BCD* is also 30° because they are formed by an angle bisector (divides an angle into two equal parts). Since angle *ABC* is 90° (right angle) and angle *BCD* is 30°, then angle *x* is 60° because there are 180° in a triangle.

$$180 - (90 + 30) = 60$$

The correct answer is C. *Always mark in diagrams as you read descriptions and information about them. This includes what you are looking for.*

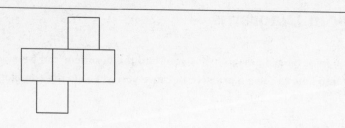

2. If each square in the figure above has a side of length 3, what is the perimeter?

    A. 12
    B. 14
    C. 21
    D. 30
    E. 36

Mark the known facts.

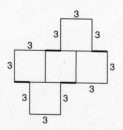

We now have a calculation for the perimeter: 30 plus the darkened part. Now look carefully at the top two darkened parts. They will add up to 3. (Notice how the top square may slide over to illustrate that fact.)

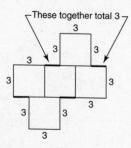

The same is true for the bottom darkened parts. They will add up to 3.

Thus, the total perimeter is 30 + 6 = 36, Choice E.

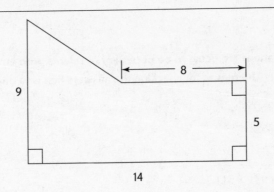

3. What is the area of the preceding figure in square units?

    A.   60
    B.   70
    C.   82
    D.   94
    E.   104

Underline or circle the words area of the figure. Since this is an irregular figure, use common shapes to work it out.

Start by finding the area of the rectangle, which is length times width.

$$14 \times 5 = 70$$

So, the area of the rectangle is 70 square units. At this point, you can eliminate choices A and B. The area must be greater than 70.

Now, you need to find the dimensions of the triangle. By using the dimensions given and subtracting from the length, you get the following dimensions:

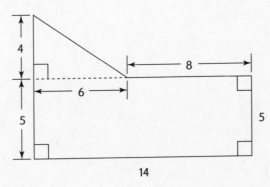

You only need the base and height of the triangle to find the area. The height is 4 and the base is 6.

$$A = \tfrac{1}{2} bh$$
$$A = \tfrac{1}{2}(6)(4)$$
$$A = \tfrac{1}{2}(24) = 12$$

Now add the areas of the rectangle and triangle, $70 + 12 = 82$. The correct answer is C.

Approximate

If it appears that extensive calculations are going to be necessary to solve a problem, check to see how far apart the choices are and then approximate. The reason for checking the answers first is to give you a guide to how freely you can approximate.

Sample

1. Which is the best estimate of 931×311?

A.   2,700
B.   27,000
C.   270,000
D.   2,700,000
E.   27,000,000

First, check the answer choices to see how far apart they are. This gives you an indication of how close your approximation should be. In this case, the choices are far apart, so your approximation does not need to be too accurate. As a matter of fact, these choices differ only by the number of zeros after 27. So be careful that you have the correct number of zeros in your estimate.

Round each number to the nearest hundred.

$$932 \times 311$$
$$\downarrow \qquad \downarrow$$
$$900 \times 300 = 270,000$$

So the best estimate is 270,000. The correct answer is C.

PART II

MATH REVIEW

A Quick Review of Mathematics

The following pages are designed to give you a quick review of some of the basic skills used on the ELM. Before beginning the diagnostic review tests, it is wise to become familiar with basic mathematics terminology, formulas, and general mathematical information. These topics are covered first in this chapter. Then proceed to the arithmetic diagnostic test, which you should take to spot your weak areas. Then use the arithmetic review that follows to strengthen those areas.

After reviewing the arithmetic, take the algebra diagnostic test and again use the review that follows to strengthen your weak areas. Next, take the geometry diagnostic test and carefully read the complete geometry review.

Even if you are strong in arithmetic, algebra, and geometry, you might wish to skim the topic headings in each area to refresh your memory about important concepts. If you are weak in math, you should read through the complete review.

Symbols, Terminology, Formulas, and General Mathematical Information

Common Math Symbols and Terms

Symbol References:

=	is equal to
≠	is not equal to
≈	is approximately equal to
>	is greater than
<	is less than
≥	is greater than or equal to
≤	is less than or equal to
‖	is parallel to
⊥	is perpendicular to

Terms:

Natural numbers	The counting numbers: 1, 2, 3, . . .
Whole numbers	The counting numbers beginning with zero: 0, 1, 2, 3, . . .
Integers	Positive and negative whole numbers and zero: . . . −3, −2, −1, 0, 1, 2, . . .
Odd number	Number not divisible by 2: 1, 3, 5, 7, . . .
Even number	Number divisible by 2: 0, 2, 4, 6, . . .
Prime number	Number divisible by only 1 and itself: 2, 3, 5, 7, 11, 13, . . .
Composite number	Number divisible by more than just 1 and itself: 4, 6, 8, 9, 10, 12, 14, 15, . . . (0 and 1 are neither prime nor composite)

Terms:	
Square	The results when a number is multiplied by itself: $2 \times 2 = 4$; $3 \times 3 = 9$. Examples of squares are 1, 4, 9, 16, 25, 36, . . .
Cube	The results when a number is multiplied by itself twice: $2 \times 2 \times 2 = 8$; $3 \times 3 \times 3 = 27$. Examples of cubes are 1, 8, 27, 64 . . .

Math Formulas

Triangle	Perimeter = $s_1 + s_2 + s_3$ Area = $\frac{1}{2} bh$
Square	Perimeter = $4s$ Area = $s \times s$ or s^2
Rectangle	Perimeter = $2(b + h)$, or $2b + 2h$ Area = bh, or lw
Parallelogram	Perimeter = $2(l + w)$, or $2l + 2w$ Area = bh
Trapezoid	Perimeter = $b_1 + b_2 + s_1 + s_2$ Area = $\frac{1}{2} h (b_1 + b_2)$, or $h\left(\dfrac{b_1 + b_2}{2}\right)$
Circle	Circumference = $2\pi r$ or πd Area = πr^2
Cube	Volume = $s \cdot s \cdot s = s^3$ Surface area = $s \cdot s \cdot 6$
Rectangular Prism	Volume = $l \cdot w \cdot h$ Surface area = $2(lw) + 2(lh) + 2(wh)$

Pythagorean theorem ($a^2 + b^2 = c^2$): The sum of the square of the legs of a right triangle equals the square of the hypotenuse.

Important Equivalents

$$\frac{1}{100} = 0.1 = 1\%$$

$$\frac{1}{10} = .1 = .10 = 10\%$$

$$\frac{1}{5} = \frac{2}{10} = .2 = .20 = 20\%$$

$$\frac{3}{10} = .3 = .30 = 30\%$$

$$\frac{2}{5} = \frac{4}{10} = .4 = .40 = 40\%$$

$$\frac{1}{2} = \frac{5}{10} = .5 = .50 = 50\%$$

$$\frac{3}{5} = \frac{6}{10} = .6 = .60 = 60\%$$

$$\frac{7}{10} = .7 = .70 = 70\%$$

$$\frac{4}{5} = \frac{8}{10} = .8 = .80 = 80\%$$

$$\frac{9}{10} = .9 = .90 = 90\%$$

$$\frac{1}{4} = \frac{25}{100} = .25 = 25\%$$

$$\frac{3}{4} = \frac{75}{100} = .75 = 75\%$$

$$\frac{1}{3} = .33\frac{1}{3} = 33\frac{1}{3}\%$$

$$\frac{2}{3} = .66\frac{2}{3} = 66\frac{2}{3}\%$$

$$\frac{1}{8} = .125 = .12\frac{1}{2} = 12\frac{1}{2}\%$$

$$\frac{3}{8} = .375 = .37\frac{1}{2} = 37\frac{1}{2}\%$$

$$\frac{5}{8} = .625 = .62\frac{1}{2} = 62\frac{1}{2}\%$$

$$\frac{7}{8} = .875 = .87\frac{1}{2} = 87\frac{1}{2}\%$$

$$\frac{1}{6} = .16\frac{2}{3} = 16\frac{2}{3}\%$$

$$\frac{5}{6} = .83\frac{1}{3} = 83\frac{1}{3}\%$$

$$1 = 1.00 = 100\%$$

$$2 = 2.00 = 200\%$$

$$3\frac{1}{2} = 3.5 = 3.50 = 350\%$$

Math Words and Phrases

Words that signal an operation:

Addition

- Sum
- Total
- Plus
- Increase
- More than
- Greater than

Multiplication

- Of
- Product
- Times
- At (sometimes)
- Total (sometimes)

Subtraction

- Difference
- Less
- Decreased
- Reduced
- Fewer
- Have left

Division

- Quotient
- Divisor
- Dividend
- Ratio
- Parts

Mathematical Properties

Some Properties (Axioms) of Addition

Commutative means that the *order* does not make any difference.

$$2 + 3 = 3 + 2$$
$$a + b = b + a$$

Note: The commutative property does *not* hold for subtraction.

$$3 - 1 \neq 1 - 3$$
$$a - b \neq b - a$$

Associative means that the *grouping* does not make any difference.

$$(2 + 3) + 4 = 2 + (3 + 4)$$
$$(a + b) + c = a + (b + c)$$

The grouping has changed (parentheses moved), but the sides are still equal.

Note: The associative property does *not* hold for subtraction.

$$4 - (3 - 1) \neq (4 - 3) - 1$$
$$a - (b - c) \neq (a - b) - c$$

The *identity element* for addition is 0. Any number added to 0 gives the original number.

$$3 + 0 = 3$$
$$a + 0 = a$$

The *additive inverse* is the opposite (negative) of the number. Any number plus its additive inverse equals 0 (the identity).

$3 + (-3) = 0$; therefore, 3 and -3 are inverses.

$-2 + 2 = 0$; therefore, -2 and 2 are inverses.

$a + (-a) = 0$; therefore, a and $-a$ are inverses.

Some Properties (Axioms) of Multiplication

Commutative means that the *order* does not make any difference.

$2 \times 3 = 3 \times 2$

$a \times b = b \times a$

Note: The commutative property does *not* hold for division.

$2 \div 4 \neq 4 \div 2$

Associative means that the *grouping* does not make any difference.

$(2 \times 3) \times 4 = 2 \times (3 \times 4)$

$(a \times b) \times c = a \times (b \times c)$

The grouping has changed (parentheses moved), but the sides are still equal.

Note: The associative property does *not* hold for division.

$(8 \div 4) \div 2 \neq 8 \div (4 \div 2)$

The *identity element* for multiplication is 1. Any number multiplied by 1 gives the original number.

$3 \times 1 = 3$

$a \times 1 = a$

The *multiplicative inverse* is the reciprocal of the number. Any number multiplied by its reciprocal equals 1.

$2 \times \frac{1}{2} = 1$; therefore, 2 and $\frac{1}{2}$ are inverses.

$a \times \frac{1}{a} = 1$; therefore, a and $\frac{1}{a}$ are inverses.

A Property of Two Operations

The *distributive property* is the process of distributing the number on the outside of a set of parentheses to each number on the inside.

$2(3 + 4) = 2(3) + 2(4)$

$a(b + c) = a(b) + a(c)$

Note: You cannot use the distributive property with only one operation.

$3(4 \times 5 \times 6) \neq 3(4) \times 3(5) \times 3(6)$

$a(bcd) \neq a(b) \times a(c) \times a(d)$ or $(ab)(ac)(ad)$

Arithmetic Diagnostic Test

Questions

1. 28×39 is approximately:

2. $6 = \frac{?}{4}$

3. Change $5\frac{3}{4}$ to an improper fraction.

4. Change $\frac{32}{6}$ to a whole number or mixed number in lowest terms.

5. $\frac{2}{5} + \frac{3}{5} =$

6. $1\frac{3}{8} + 2\frac{5}{6} =$

7. $\frac{7}{9} - \frac{5}{9} =$

8. $11 - \frac{2}{3} =$

9. $6\frac{1}{4} - 3\frac{3}{4} =$

10. $\frac{1}{6} \times \frac{1}{6} =$

11. $2\frac{3}{8} \times 1\frac{5}{6} =$

12. $\frac{1}{4} \div \frac{3}{2} =$

13. $2\frac{3}{7} \div 1\frac{1}{4} =$

14. $.07 + 1.2 + .471 =$

15. $.45 - .003 =$

16. $\$78.24 - \$31.68 =$

17. $.5 \times .5 =$

18. $8.001 \times 2.3 =$

19. $.7\overline{)\,.147} =$

20. $.002\overline{)\,12} =$

21. $\frac{1}{3}$ of $7.20 =

22. Circle the larger number: 7.9 or 4.35.

23. 39 out of 100 means:

24. Change 4% to a decimal.

25. 46% of 58 =

26. Change .009 to a percent.

27. Change 12.5% to a fraction.

28. Change $\frac{3}{8}$ to a percent.

29. Is 93 prime?

30. What is the percent increase in a rise in temperature from 80° to 100°?

31. $-6 + 8 =$

32. $-7 \times -9 =$

33. $|-9| =$

34. $8^2 =$

35. $3^2 \times 3^5 =$

36. The square root of 30 is approximately equal to:

37. What is the median of the numbers 4, 3, 5, 7, 9, and 1?

38. Based on the following circle graph, how much time does Timmy spend doing homework?

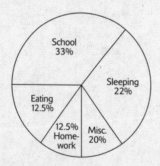

How Timmy Spends His 24-Hour Day

Answers

1. 1,200

2. 24

3. $\frac{23}{4}$

4. $5\frac{2}{6}$ or $5\frac{1}{3}$

5. $\frac{5}{5}$ or 1

6. $4\frac{5}{24}$

7. $\frac{2}{9}$

8. $10\frac{1}{3}$

9. $2\frac{2}{4}$ or $2\frac{1}{2}$

10. $\frac{1}{36}$

11. $\frac{209}{48}$ or $4\frac{17}{48}$

12. $\frac{1}{6}$

13. $\frac{68}{35}$ or $1\frac{33}{35}$

14. 1.741

15. .447

16. $46.56

17. .25

18. 18.4023

19. .21

20. 6,000

21. $2.40

22. 7.9

23. 39% or $\frac{39}{100}$

24. .04

25. 26.68

26. .9% or $\frac{9}{10}$%

27. $\frac{125}{1000}$ or $\frac{1}{8}$

28. 37.5% or $37\frac{1}{2}$%

29. No.

30. 25%

31. 2

32. 63

33. 9

34. 64

35. 3^7

36. 5.5 or $5\frac{1}{2}$

37. $4\frac{1}{2}$ or 4.5

38. 3 hours

Arithmetic Review

Place Value

Each position in any number has *place value*. For instance, in the number 485, 4 is in the hundreds place, 8 is in the tens place, and 5 is in the ones place. Thus, place value is as follows:

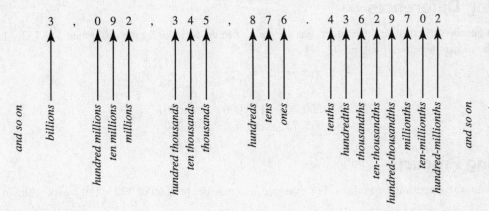

Rounding Off

To round off any number:

1. Underline the place value to which you're rounding off.
2. Look to the immediate right (one place) of your underlined place value.
3. Identify the number (the one to the right). If it is 5 or higher, round your underlined place value up 1. If the number (the one to the right) is 4 or less, leave your underlined place value as it is and change all the other numbers to its right to zeros. For example:

Round to the nearest thousand:

345,678 becomes 346,000

928,499 becomes 928,000

This works with decimals as well. Round to the nearest hundredth:

3.4678 becomes 3.47

298,435.083 becomes 298,435.08

Estimating Sums, Differences, Products, and Quotients

Knowing how to approximate or estimate not only saves you time but can also help you check your answer to determine whether it is reasonable.

Estimating Sums

Use rounded numbers to estimate sums. For example, give an estimate for the sum 3,741 + 5,021 rounded to the nearest thousand.

$$3,741 + 5,021$$
$$\downarrow \qquad \downarrow$$
$$4,000 + 5,000 = 9,000$$
So $\qquad 3,741 + 5,021 \approx 9,000$

Note: The symbol $\approx$ means is approximately equal to.

Estimating Differences

Use rounded numbers to estimate differences. For example, give an estimate for the difference $317,753 - 115,522$ rounded to the nearest hundred thousand.

$$317,753 - 115,522$$
$$\downarrow \qquad \downarrow$$
$$300,000 - 100,000 = 200,000$$
So $\qquad 317,753 - 115,522 \approx 200,000$

Estimating Products

Use rounded numbers to estimate products. For example, estimate the product of 722×489 by rounding to the nearest hundred.

$$722 \times 489$$
$$\downarrow \qquad \downarrow$$
$$700 \times 500 = 350,000$$
So $\qquad 722 \times 489 \approx 350,000$

If both multipliers end in 50 or are halfway numbers, then rounding one number up and one number down gives a better estimate of the product. For example, estimate the product of 650×350 by rounding to the nearest hundred.

$$650 \times 350$$
$$\downarrow \qquad \downarrow$$
Round one number up and one down. $\quad 700 \times 300 = 210,000$
So $\qquad\qquad\qquad\qquad\qquad 650 \times 300 \approx 210,000$

You can also round the first number down and the second number up and get this estimate:

$$650 \times 350$$
$$\downarrow \qquad \downarrow$$
$$600 \times 400 = 240,000$$
So $\qquad 650 \times 350 \approx 240,000$

In either case, this approximation is closer than if you round both numbers up, which is the standard rule.

Estimating Quotients

Use rounded numbers to estimate quotients. For example, estimate the quotient of $891 \div 288$ by rounding to the nearest hundred.

$$891 \div 288$$
$$\downarrow \qquad \downarrow$$
$$900 \div 300 = 3$$
So $\qquad 891 \div 288 = 3$

Fractions

Fractions consist of two numbers: a *numerator* (which is above the line) and a *denominator* (which is below the line).

$$\frac{1}{2} \frac{\text{numerator}}{\text{denominator}} \quad \text{or} \quad \text{numerator } \frac{1}{2} \text{ denominator}$$

The denominator indicates the number of equal parts into which something is divided. The numerator indicates how many of these equal parts are contained in the fraction. Thus, if the fraction is $\frac{3}{5}$ of a pie, then the denominator, 5, indicates that the pie has been divided into 5 equal parts, of which 3 (the numerator) are in the fraction.

Sometimes it helps to think of the dividing line (in the middle of a fraction) as meaning *out of*. In other words, $\frac{3}{5}$ also means 3 *out of* 5 equal pieces from the whole pie.

Common Fractions and Improper Fractions

A fraction like $\frac{3}{5}$, where the numerator is smaller than the denominator, is less than 1. This kind of fraction is called a *common fraction*.

Sometimes a fraction represents more than 1. This is when the numerator is larger than the denominator. Thus, $\frac{12}{7}$ is more than 1. This is called an *improper fraction*.

Mixed Numbers

When a term contains both a whole number (such as 3, 8, or 25) and a fraction (such as $\frac{1}{2}$, $\frac{1}{4}$, or $\frac{3}{4}$), it is called a *mixed number*. For example, $5\frac{1}{4}$ and $290\frac{3}{4}$ are both mixed numbers.

To change an improper fraction to a mixed number, divide the denominator into the numerator. For example:

$$\frac{18}{5} = 3\frac{3}{5} \qquad 5\overline{)18} \begin{array}{l} 3 \\ \underline{15} \\ 3 \end{array}$$

To change a mixed number to an improper fraction, multiply the denominator by the whole number, add the numerator and put the total over the original denominator. For example:

$$4\frac{1}{2} = \frac{9}{2} \qquad 2 \times 4 + 1 = 9$$

Reducing Fractions

A fraction must be reduced to *lowest terms*. This is done by dividing both the numerator and the denominator by the largest number that divides evenly into both. For example, $\frac{14}{16}$ is reduced by dividing both terms by 2, giving $\frac{7}{8}$. Likewise, $\frac{20}{25}$ is reduced to $\frac{4}{5}$ by dividing both the numerator and denominator by 5.

Adding Fractions

To add fractions, first change all denominators to their *lowest common denominator* (LCD)—the lowest number that can be divided evenly by all the denominators in the problem. When all the denominators are the same, add fractions by simply adding the numerators (the denominator remains the same). For example:

$$\begin{array}{r} \frac{3}{8} = \frac{3}{8} \\ +\frac{1}{2} = \frac{4}{8} \\ \hline \frac{7}{8} \end{array} \quad \left\{ \begin{array}{l} \text{one-half is} \\ \text{changed to} \\ \text{four-eighths} \end{array} \right. \qquad \begin{array}{r} \frac{1}{4} = \frac{3}{12} \\ +\frac{1}{3} = \frac{4}{12} \\ \hline \frac{7}{12} \end{array} \quad \left\{ \begin{array}{l} \text{change both} \\ \text{fractions to} \\ \text{LCD of 12} \end{array} \right.$$

43

In the first example, we changed the $\frac{1}{2}$ to $\frac{4}{8}$ because 8 is the LCD, and then we added the numerators 3 and 4 to get $\frac{7}{8}$. In the second example, we had to change both fractions to get the LCD of 12, and then we added the numerators to get $\frac{7}{12}$. Of course, if the denominators are already the same, just add the numerators. For example:

$$\frac{6}{11} + \frac{3}{11} = \frac{9}{11}$$

Adding Mixed Numbers

To add mixed numbers, the same rule (find the LCD) applies, but always add the whole number to get your final answer. For example:

$$2\frac{1}{2} = 2\frac{2}{4} \quad \longleftarrow \left\{ \begin{array}{l}\text{change one-half}\\ \text{to two-fourths}\end{array}\right.$$
$$+ \;\; 3\frac{1}{4} = 3\frac{1}{4}$$
$$\overline{\qquad\qquad 5\frac{3}{4}}$$
$$\longleftarrow \left\{ \begin{array}{l}\text{remember to add}\\ \text{the whole numbers}\end{array}\right.$$

Subtracting Fractions

To subtract fractions, the same rule (find the LCD) applies, except subtract the numerators. For example:

$$\frac{7}{8} = \frac{7}{8} \qquad\qquad \frac{3}{4} = \frac{9}{12}$$
$$-\frac{1}{4} = \frac{2}{8} \qquad\qquad -\frac{1}{3} = \frac{4}{12}$$
$$\overline{\quad\;\; \frac{5}{8}} \qquad\qquad \overline{\quad\;\; \frac{5}{12}}$$

Subtracting Mixed Numbers

When you subtract mixed numbers, sometimes you have to borrow from the whole number, just like you sometimes borrow from the next column when subtracting ordinary numbers. For example:

$$6\overset{4}{\cancel{5}}\overset{11}{1} \qquad\qquad\qquad 4\overset{3\frac{7}{6}}{\frac{1}{6}}$$
$$-\;129 \qquad\qquad\qquad -\;2\frac{5}{6}$$
$$\overline{\quad 522} \qquad\qquad\qquad \overline{\quad 1\frac{2}{6} = 1\frac{1}{3}}$$

$$\begin{array}{ll}\text{you borrowed 1} & \text{you borrowed one in} \\ \text{from the 10's} & \text{the form } \frac{6}{6} \text{ from} \\ \text{column} & \text{the 1's column}\end{array}$$

To subtract a mixed number from a whole number, you have to borrow from the whole number. For example:

$$6 \;\;\; = 5\frac{5}{5} \quad \longleftarrow \left\{ \begin{array}{l}\text{borrow one in the form of}\\ \frac{5}{5} \text{ from the 6}\end{array}\right.$$
$$-3\frac{1}{5} \;\; = 3\frac{1}{5}$$
$$\overline{\qquad\quad 2\frac{4}{5}}$$
$$\longleftarrow \left\{ \begin{array}{l}\text{remember to subtract the}\\ \text{remaining whole numbers}\end{array}\right.$$

Multiplying Fractions

Simply multiply the numerators, and then multiply the denominators. Reduce to lowest terms if necessary. For example:

$$\frac{2}{3} \times \frac{5}{12} = \frac{10}{36} \qquad \text{reduce } \frac{10}{36} \text{ to } \frac{5}{18}$$

This answer had to be reduced because it wasn't in lowest terms.

Canceling When Multiplying Fractions

You could have *canceled* first. Canceling eliminates the need to reduce your answer. To cancel, find a number that divides evenly into one numerator and one denominator. In this case, 2 divides evenly into 2 in the numerator (it goes in one time) and 12 in the denominator (it goes in 6 times). Thus:

$$\frac{\cancel{2}^{1}}{3} \times \frac{5}{\cancel{12}_{6}} =$$

Now that you've canceled, you can multiply as before.

$$\frac{\cancel{2}^{1}}{3} \times \frac{5}{\cancel{12}_{6}} = \frac{5}{18}$$

You can cancel only when *multiplying* fractions.

Multiplying Mixed Numbers

To multiply mixed numbers, first change any mixed number to an improper fraction. Then multiply as previously shown. To change mixed numbers to improper fractions:

1. Multiply the whole number by the denominator of the fraction.
2. Add this to the numerator of the fraction.
3. This is now your numerator.
4. The denominator remains the same.

$$3\frac{1}{3} \times 2\frac{1}{4} = \frac{10}{3} \times \frac{9}{4} = \frac{90}{12} = 7\frac{6}{12} = 7\frac{1}{2}$$

Then, change the answer, if it is in improper form, back to a mixed number and reduce if necessary.

Dividing Fractions

To divide fractions, invert (turn upside down) the second fraction and multiply. Then, reduce if necessary. For example:

$$\frac{1}{6} \div \frac{1}{5} = \frac{1}{6} \times \frac{5}{1} = \frac{5}{6} \qquad\qquad \frac{1}{6} \div \frac{1}{3} = \frac{1}{6} \times \frac{3}{1} = \frac{1}{2}$$

Simplifying Fractions

If either numerator or denominator consists of several numbers, these numbers must be combined into one number. Then, reduce if necessary. For example:

$$\frac{28 + 14}{26 + 17} = \frac{42}{43} \text{ or}$$

$$\frac{\frac{1}{4} + \frac{1}{2}}{\frac{1}{3} + \frac{1}{4}} = \frac{\frac{1}{4} + \frac{2}{4}}{\frac{4}{12} + \frac{3}{12}} = \frac{\frac{3}{4}}{\frac{7}{12}} = \frac{3}{4} \times \frac{12}{7} = \frac{36}{28} = \frac{9}{7} = 1\frac{2}{7}$$

Decimals

Fractions can also be written in decimal form by using a symbol called a *decimal point*. All numbers to the left of the decimal point are whole numbers. All numbers to the right of the decimal point are fractions with denominators of only 10, 100, 1,000, 10,000, and so on, as follows:

$$.6 = \frac{6}{10} = \frac{3}{5}$$

$$.7 = \frac{7}{10}$$

$$.07 = \frac{7}{100}$$

$$.007 = \frac{7}{1000}$$

$$.0007 = \frac{7}{10000}$$

$$.25 = \frac{25}{100} = \frac{1}{4}$$

Adding and Subtracting Decimals

To add or subtract decimals, just line up the decimal points and then add or subtract in the same manner as when adding or subtracting regular numbers. For example:

23.6 + 1.75 + 300.002 =

$$\begin{array}{r} 23.6 \\ 1.75 \\ +\,300.002 \\ \hline 325.352 \end{array}$$

Adding zeros can make the problem easier to work:

$$\begin{array}{r} 23.600 \\ 1.750 \\ +\,300.002 \\ \hline 325.352 \end{array}$$

and
54.26 − 1.1 =

$$\begin{array}{r} 54.26 \\ -\,1.10 \\ \hline 53.16 \end{array}$$

and
78.9 − 37.43 =

$$\begin{array}{r} 78.\overset{8}{\cancel{9}}{}^{1}0 \\ -\,37.43 \\ \hline 41.47 \end{array}$$

Whole numbers can have decimal points to their right. For example:

17 − 8.43 =

$$\begin{array}{r} 1\overset{6}{7}.\overset{9}{\cancel{0}}{}^{1}0 \\ -\,8.43 \\ \hline 8.57 \end{array}$$

Multiplying Decimals

To multiply decimals, multiply as usual. Then, count the total number of digits above the line that are to the right of all decimal points. Place the decimal point in the answer so that the number of digits to the right of the decimal is the same as it is above the line. For example:

$$40.012 \leftarrow \text{3 digits} \quad \left\{ \begin{array}{l} \text{total of 4 digits above the line that} \\ \text{are to the right of the decimal point} \end{array} \right.$$

$$\underline{\times \quad 3.1} \leftarrow \text{1 digit}$$

$$40012$$

$$\underline{120036}$$

$$124.0372 \leftarrow \text{4 digits} \quad \left\{ \begin{array}{l} \text{decimal point placed so there is} \\ \text{same number of digits to the right} \\ \text{of the decimal point} \end{array} \right.$$

Dividing Decimals

Dividing decimals is the same as dividing other numbers, except that when the *divisor* (the number you're dividing by) has a decimal, move it to the right as many places as necessary until it is a whole number. Then move the decimal point in the *dividend* (the number being divided into) the same number of places. Sometimes you have to add zeros to the *dividend* (the number inside the division sign).

$$1.25\overline{)5.} = 125\overline{)500.}^{\,4.}$$

or

$$0.002\overline{)26.} = 2\overline{)26000}^{\,13000}$$

Conversions

Changing Decimals to Percents

To change decimals to percents:

1. Move the decimal point two places to the right.
2. Insert a percent sign.

$$.75 = 75\%$$
$$.05 = 5\%$$

Changing Percents to Decimals

To change percents to decimals:

1. Eliminate the percent sign.
2. Move the decimal point two places to the left. (Sometimes adding zeros is necessary.)

$$75\% = .75$$
$$5\% = .05$$
$$23\% = .23$$
$$.2\% = .002$$

Changing Fractions to Percents

To change a fraction to a percent:

1. Multiply by 100.
2. Insert a percent sign.

$$\frac{1}{2} = \left(\frac{1}{2}\right) \times 100 = \frac{100}{2} = 50\%$$

$$\frac{2}{5} = \left(\frac{2}{5}\right) \times 100 = \frac{200}{5} = 40\%$$

Changing Percents to Fractions

To change percents to fractions:

1. Divide the percent by 100.
2. Eliminate the percent sign.
3. Reduce if necessary.

$$60\% = \frac{60}{100} = \frac{3}{5} \qquad 13\% = \frac{13}{100}$$

Changing Fractions to Decimals

To change a fraction to a decimal, simply do what the operation says. In other words, $\frac{13}{20}$ means 13 divided by 20. So, do just that. (Insert decimal points and zeros accordingly.)

$$20\overline{)13.00}^{.65} = .65 \qquad \frac{5}{8} = 8\overline{)5.000}^{.625} = .625$$

Changing Decimals to Fractions

To change a decimal to a fraction:

1. Move the decimal point two places to the right.
2. Put that number over 100.
3. Reduce if necessary.

$$.65 = \frac{65}{100} = \frac{13}{20}$$
$$.05 = \frac{5}{100} = \frac{1}{20}$$
$$.75 = \frac{75}{100} = \frac{3}{4}$$

Read it: .8

Write it: $\frac{8}{10}$

Reduce it: $\frac{4}{5}$

Using Percents

Finding the Percent of a Number

To determine the percent of a number, change the percent to a fraction or decimal (whichever is easier for you) and multiply. The word *of* means multiply.

For example:

1. What is 20% of 80?

$$\left(\frac{20}{100}\right) \times 80 = \frac{1600}{100} = 16 \text{ or } .20 \times 80 = 16.00 = 16$$

2. What is 12% of 50?

$$\left(\frac{12}{100}\right) \times 50 = \frac{600}{100} = 6 \text{ or } .12 \times 50 = 6.00 = 6$$

3. What is $\frac{1}{2}$% of 18?

$$\frac{\frac{1}{2}}{100} \times 18 = \left(\frac{1}{200}\right) \times 18 = \frac{18}{200} = \frac{9}{100} \text{ or } .005 \times 18 = .09$$

Other Applications of Percent

Turn the question (word for word) into an equation. For what substitute the letter *x;* for *is* substitute an *equal sign;* for *of* substitute a *multiplication sign.* Change percents to decimals or fractions, whichever you find easier. Then solve the equation.

For example:

1. 18 is what percent of 90?

$$18 = x(90)$$
$$\frac{18}{90} = x$$
$$\frac{1}{5} = x$$
$$20\% = x$$

2. 10 is 50% of what number?

$$10 = .50(x)$$
$$\frac{10}{.50} = x$$
$$20 = x$$

3. What is 15% of 60?

$$x = \left(\frac{15}{100}\right) \times 60 = \frac{900}{100} = 9$$

$$\text{or } .15(60) = 9$$

Percentage Increase or Decrease

To find the *percentage change* (increase or decrease), use this formula:

$$\frac{\text{change}}{\text{starting point}} \times 100 = \text{percentage change}$$

For example:

1. What is the percentage decrease of a $500 item on sale for $400?

$$\text{Change: } 500 - 400 = 100$$

$$\frac{\text{change}}{\text{starting point}} \times 100 = \frac{100}{500} \times 100 = \frac{1}{5} \times 100 = 20\% \text{ decrease}$$

2. What is the percentage increase of Jon's salary if it goes from $150 a month to $200 a month?

$$\text{Change: } 200 - 150 = 50$$

$$\frac{\text{change}}{\text{starting point}} \times 100 = \frac{50}{150} \times 100 = \frac{1}{3} \times 100 = 33\frac{1}{3}\% \text{ increase}$$

Signed Numbers (Positive Numbers and Negative Numbers)

On a number line, numbers to the right of 0 are positive. Numbers to the left of 0 are negative, as follows:

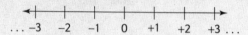

$$\ldots -3 \quad -2 \quad -1 \quad 0 \quad +1 \quad +2 \quad +3 \ldots$$

Given any two numbers on a number line, the one on the right is always larger, regardless of its sign (positive or negative).

Adding Signed Numbers

When adding two numbers with the same sign (either both positive or both negative), add the numbers and keep the same sign. For example:

$$\begin{array}{r} +5 \\ ++7 \\ \hline +12 \end{array} \qquad \begin{array}{r} -8 \\ +-3 \\ \hline -11 \end{array}$$

When adding two numbers with different signs (one positive and one negative), subtract the numbers and keep the sign from the larger one. For example:

$$\begin{array}{r} +5 \\ +-7 \\ \hline -2 \end{array} \qquad \begin{array}{r} -59 \\ ++72 \\ \hline +13 \end{array}$$

Subtracting Signed Numbers

To subtract positive and/or negative numbers, just change the sign of the number being subtracted and add. For example:

$$\begin{array}{r} +12 \\ -+4 \end{array} \quad \begin{array}{r} +12 \\ +-4 \\ \hline +8 \end{array} \qquad \begin{array}{r} -19 \\ -+6 \end{array} \quad \begin{array}{r} -19 \\ +-6 \\ \hline -25 \end{array}$$

$$\begin{array}{r} -14 \\ --4 \end{array} \quad \begin{array}{r} -14 \\ ++4 \\ \hline -10 \end{array} \qquad \begin{array}{r} +20 \\ --3 \end{array} \quad \begin{array}{r} +20 \\ ++3 \\ \hline +23 \end{array}$$

Multiplying and Dividing Signed Numbers

To multiply or divide signed numbers, treat them just like regular numbers but remember this rule: An odd number of negative signs produces a negative answer; an even number of negative signs produces a positive answer. For example:

$$(-3)(+8)(-5)(-1)(-2) = +240$$

Absolute Value

The numerical value when direction or sign is not considered is called the *absolute value*. The value of a number is written $|3| = 3$ and $|-4| = 4$. The absolute value of a number is always positive except when the number is 0. For example:

$$|-8| = 8$$
$$|3 - 9| = |-6| = 6$$
$$3 - |-6| = 3 - 6 = -3$$

Note: Absolute values must be taken first, or the work must be done first within the absolute value signs.

Powers and Exponents

An *exponent* is a positive or negative number placed above and to the right of a quantity. It expresses the power to which the quantity is to be raised or lowered. In 4^3, 3 is the exponent. It shows that 4 is to be used as a factor three times. $4 \times 4 \times 4$ (multiplied by itself twice). 4^3 is read *four to the third power* (or *four cubed*). For example:

$$2^4 = 2 \times 2 \times 2 \times 2 = 16$$
$$3^2 = 3 \times 3 = 9$$

Remember that $x^1 = x$ and $x^0 = 1$ when x is any number (other than 0). For example:

$$2^1 = 2$$
$$2^0 = 1$$
$$3^1 = 3$$
$$3^0 = 1$$

Negative Exponents

If an exponent is negative, such as 3^{-2}, then the number and exponent can be dropped under the number 1 in a fraction to remove the negative sign. The number can be simplified as follows:

$$3^{-2} = \frac{1}{3^2} = \frac{1}{9}$$

Operations with Powers and Exponents

To multiply two numbers with exponents, if the base numbers are the same, simply keep the base number and add the exponents. For example:

$$2^3 \times 2^5 = 2^8 \qquad [(2 \times 2 \times 2) \times (2 \times 2 \times 2 \times 2 \times 2) = 2^8] \qquad [2^{(3+5)} = 2^8]$$
$$7^2 \times 7^4 = 7^6$$

To divide two numbers with exponents, if the base numbers are the same, simply keep the base number and subtract the second exponent from the first. For example:

$$3^4 \div 3^2 = 3^2 \qquad \left[3^{(4-2)} = 3^2\right]$$
$$\frac{9^6}{9^2} = 9^6 \div 9^2 = 9^4 \qquad \left[9^{(6-2)} = 9^4\right]$$

Three Notes:

- If the base numbers are different in multiplication or division, simplify each number with an exponent first, and then perform the operation.
- To add or subtract numbers with exponents, whether the base is the same or different, simplify each number with an exponent first, and then perform the indicated operation.
- If a number with an exponent is taken to another power $(4^2)^3$, simply keep the original base number and multiply the exponents. For example:

$$(4^2)^3 = 4^6 \qquad [4^{(2 \times 3)} = 4^6]$$
$$(3^4)^2 = 3^8$$

Squares and Square Roots

To *square* a number, just multiply it by itself. For example, 6 squared (written 6^2) is 6×6, or 36. Thirty-six is called a *perfect square* (the square of a whole number).

Following is a list of some perfect squares:

$$1^2 = 1$$
$$2^2 = 4$$
$$3^2 = 9$$
$$4^2 = 16$$
$$5^2 = 25$$
$$6^2 = 36$$
$$7^2 = 49$$
$$8^2 = 64$$
$$9^2 = 81$$
$$10^2 = 100$$
$$11^2 = 121$$
$$12^2 = 144 \ldots$$

Square roots of nonperfect squares can be approximated. Two approximations to remember are:

$$\sqrt{2} \approx 1.4$$
$$\sqrt{3} \approx 1.7$$

To find the *square root* of a number, find some number that when multiplied by itself gives you the original number. In other words, to find the square root of 25, find the number that when multiplied by itself gives you 25. The square root of 25, then, is 5. The symbol for square root is $\sqrt{}$. Following is a list of perfect (whole number) square roots:

$$\sqrt{1} = 1$$
$$\sqrt{4} = 2$$
$$\sqrt{9} = 3$$
$$\sqrt{16} = 4$$
$$\sqrt{25} = 5$$
$$\sqrt{36} = 6$$
$$\sqrt{49} = 7$$
$$\sqrt{64} = 8$$
$$\sqrt{81} = 9$$
$$\sqrt{100} = 10$$

Square Root Rules

Two numbers multiplied under a radical (square root) sign equal the product of the two square roots. For example:

$$\sqrt{(4)(25)} = \sqrt{4} \times \sqrt{25} = 2 \times 5 = 10 \ \text{ or } \ \sqrt{100} = 10$$

Likewise with division:

$$\sqrt{\frac{64}{4}} = \frac{\sqrt{64}}{\sqrt{4}} = \frac{8}{2} = 4 \ \text{ or } \ \sqrt{16} = 4$$

Addition and subtraction, however, are different. The numbers must be combined under the radical before any computation of square roots is done. For example:

$$\sqrt{10+6} = \sqrt{16} = 4 \qquad \sqrt{10+6} \text{ does } not \text{ equal } [\neq]\sqrt{10} + \sqrt{6}$$

$$\sqrt{93-12} = \sqrt{81} = 9$$

Approximating Square Roots

To find a square root that is not a whole number, you should approximate. For example:

Approximate $\sqrt{57}$.

Since $\sqrt{57}$ is between $\sqrt{49}$ and $\sqrt{64}$, it falls somewhere between 7 and 8. And because 57 is just about halfway between 49 and 64, $\sqrt{57}$ is approximately $7\frac{1}{2}$.

Approximate $\sqrt{83}$.

$$\overset{9}{\sqrt{81}} < \sqrt{83} < \overset{10}{\sqrt{100}}$$

Since $\sqrt{83}$ is slightly more than $\sqrt{81}$ (whose square root is 9), $\sqrt{83}$ is a little more than 9. Because 83 is only two steps up from the nearest perfect square (81) and 17 steps to the next perfect square (100), 83 is $\frac{2}{19}$ of the way to 100.

$$\frac{2}{19} \approx \frac{2}{20} \approx \frac{1}{10} = .1$$

Therefore, $\sqrt{83} \approx 9.1$.

Simplifying Square Roots

To simplify numbers under a radical (square root sign):

1. Factor the number to two numbers, one (or more) of which is a perfect square.
2. Take the square root of the perfect square(s).
3. Leave the other factors under the $\sqrt{}$.

Simplify $\sqrt{75}$.

$$\sqrt{75} = \sqrt{25 \times 3} = \sqrt{25} \times \sqrt{3} = 5\sqrt{3}$$

Simplify $\sqrt{200}$

$$\sqrt{200} = \sqrt{100 \times 2} = \sqrt{100} \times \sqrt{2} = 10\sqrt{2}$$

Simplify $\sqrt{900}$.

$$\sqrt{900} = \sqrt{100 \times 9} = \sqrt{100} \times \sqrt{9} = 10 \times 3 = 30$$

Parentheses

Parentheses are used to group numbers. Everything inside a set of parentheses must be done before any other operations. For example:

$$6 - (-3 + a - 2b + c) =$$
$$6 + (+3 - a + 2b - c) =$$
$$6 + 3 - a + 2b - c = 9 - a + 2b - c$$

Order of Operations

If addition, multiplication, division, powers, parentheses, and so on are all contained in one problem, the order of operations is as follows:

1. parentheses
2. exponents

3. multiplication $\Big\}$ whichever comes first, left to right
4. division

5. addition $\Big\}$ whichever comes first, left to right
6. subtraction

For example:

$$10 - 3 \times 6 + 10^2 + (6 + 1) \times 4 =$$
$$10 - 3 \times 6 + 10^2 + (7) \times 4 = \text{(parentheses first)}$$
$$10 - 3 \times 6 + 100 + (7) \times 4 = \text{(exponents next)}$$
$$10 - 18 + 100 + 28 = \text{(multiplication)}$$
$$-8 + 100 + 28 = \text{(addition/subtraction, left to right)}$$
$$92 + 28 = 120$$

An easy way to remember the order of operations after parentheses is: Please Excuse My Dear Aunt Sally, or PEMDAS (Parentheses, Exponents, Multiplication, Division, Addition, Subtraction).

Basic Statistics

The study of numerical data and its distribution is called *statistics*.

The three basic measures indicating the center of a distribution are: *mean, median,* and *mode.*

Mean, Arithmetic Mean, or Average

To find the *average* of a group of numbers:

1. Add them up.
2. Divide by the number of items you added.

For example:

1. What is the average of 10, 20, 35, 40, and 45?

$$10 + 20 + 35 + 40 + 45 = 150$$
$$150 \div 5 = 30$$

The average is 30.

2. What is the average of 0, 12, 18, 20, 31, and 45?

$$0 + 12 + 18 + 20 + 31 + 45 = 126$$
$$126 \div 6 = 21$$

The average is 21.

3. What is the average of 25, 27, 27, and 27?

$$25 + 27 + 27 + 27 = 106$$
$$106 \div 4 = 26\frac{1}{2}$$

The average is $26\frac{1}{2}$.

Median

A *median* is simply the middle number in a list of numbers that have been written in numerical order.

For example, in the following list—3, 4, 6, 9, 21, 24, 56—the number 9 is the median. If the list contains an even number of items, average the two middle numbers to get the median.

For example, in the following list—5, 6, 7, 8, 9, 10—the median is $7\frac{1}{2}$. Because there is an even number of items, the average of the middle two, 7 and 8, gives the median. The list has to be in numerical order (or put in numerical order) first. The median is easy to calculate and is not influenced by extreme measures.

Mode

A *mode* is simply the number most frequently listed in a group of numbers.

For example, in the following group—5, 9, 7, 3, 9, 4, 6, 9, 7, 9, 2—the mode is 9 because it appears more often than any other number. There can be more than one mode. If there are two modes, the group is called *bimodal*.

Graphs

Information can be displayed in many ways. The three basic types of graphs you should know about are bar graphs, line graphs, and circle graphs (or pie charts).

When answering questions related to a graph:

- Examine the entire graph—notice labels and headings.
- Focus on the information given.
- Look for major changes—high points, low points, trends.
- Do not memorize the graph; refer to it.
- Pay special attention to the part of the graph to which the question refers.
- Reread the headings and labels if you don't understand.

Bar Graphs

Bar graphs convert the information in a chart into separate bars or columns. Some graphs list numbers along one edge and places, dates, people, or things (individual categories) along the other edge. Always try to determine the relationship between the columns in a graph or chart.

For example:

1. The following bar graph indicates that City W has approximately how many more billboards than City Y?

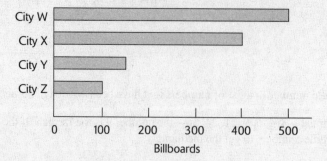

The graph shows the number of billboards in each city, with the numbers given along the bottom of the graph in increases of 100. The names are listed along the left side. City W has approximately 500 billboards. The bar graph for City Y stops about halfway between 100 and 200. Consider that halfway between 100 and 200 is 150. So City W (500) has approximately 350 more billboards than City Y (150).

$$500 - 150 = 350$$

2. Based on the following bar graph, answer these questions:

A. The number of books sold by Mystery Mystery from 1990 to 1992 exceeded the number of those sold by All Sports by approximately how many?

B. From 1991 to 1992, the percent increase in number of books sold by All Sports exceeded the percent increase in number of books sold by Mystery Mystery by approximately how much?

C. What caused the 1992 decline in Reference Unlimited's number of books sold?

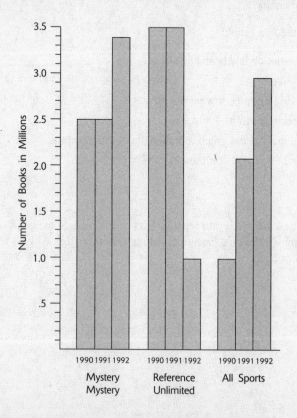

The graph contains multiple bars representing each publisher. Each single bar stands for the number of books sold in a single year. You might be tempted to write out the numbers as you do your arithmetic (3.5 million = 3,500,000). Writing out the numbers is unnecessary, as it often is with graphs that use large numbers. Since all measurements are in millions, adding zeros does not add precision to the numbers.

A. Referring to the Mystery Mystery bars, the number of books sold per year is as follows:

$$1990 = 2.5$$
$$1991 = 2.5$$
$$1992 = 3.4$$

Use a piece of paper as a straightedge to determine this last number. Totaling the number of books sold for all 3 years gives 8.4.

Referring to the All Sports bars, the number of books sold per year is as follows:

$$1990 = 1$$
$$1991 = 2.1$$
$$1992 = 3$$

Again, use a piece of paper as a straightedge, but don't designate numbers beyond the nearest 10th because the graph numbers prescribe no greater accuracy than this. Totaling the number of books sold for all 3 years gives 6.1.

So, the number of books sold by Mystery Mystery exceeded the number of books sold by All Sports by 2.3 million.

B. Graph and chart questions might ask you to calculate percent increase or percent decrease. The formula for figuring either of these is the same.

$$\frac{\text{change}}{\text{starting point}} = \text{percent change}$$

In this case, the percent increase in number of books sold by Mystery Mystery can be calculated first.

$$\text{Number of books sold in } 1991 = 2.5$$
$$\text{Number of books sold in } 1992 = 3.4$$
$$\text{Change} = .9$$

The 1991 amount is the starting point, so:

$$\frac{\text{change}}{\text{starting point}} = \frac{.9}{2.5} = 36\%$$

The percent increase in number of books sold by All Sports can be calculated as follows:

$$\text{Number of books sold in } 1991 = 2.1$$
$$\text{Number of books sold in } 1992 = 3.0$$
$$\text{Change} = .9$$

$$\frac{\text{change}}{\text{starting point}} = \frac{.9}{2.1} = 4.28 \approx 43\%$$

So the percent increase of All Sports exceeded that of Mystery Mystery by 7%:

$$43\% - 36\% = 7\%$$

C. This question cannot be answered based on the information in the graph. Never assume information that is not given. In this case, the multiple factors that could cause a decline in the number of books sold are not represented by the graph.

Line Graphs

Line graphs convert data into points on a grid. These points are then connected to show a relationship among items, dates, times, and so on. Notice the slopes of the lines connecting the points. These lines show increases and decreases— the sharper the slope *upward,* the greater the *increase,* the sharper the slope *downward,* the greater the *decrease.* Line graphs can show trends, or changes, in data over a period of time.

For example:

1. Based on the following line graph, answer these questions:

   A. In what year was the property value of Moose Lake Resort about $500,000?

   B. In which 10-year period was there the greatest decrease in the property value of Moose Lake Resort?

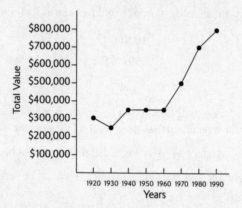

A. The information along the left side of the graph shows the property value of Moose Lake Resort in increments of $100,000. The bottom of the graph shows the years from 1920 to 1990. In 1970, the property value was about $500,000. Using a sheet of paper as a straightedge helps to see that the dot in the 1970 column lines up with $500,000 on the left.

B. Since the slope of the line goes down from 1920 to 1930, there must have been a decrease in property value. If you read the actual numbers, you notice a decrease from $300,000 to about $250,000.

2. According to the following line graph, the tomato plant grew the most between which two weeks?

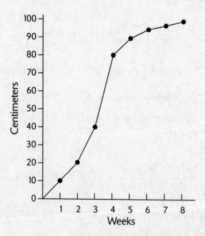

The numbers at the bottom of the graph give the weeks of growth of the plant. The numbers on the left give the height of the plant in centimeters. The sharpest upward slope occurs between week 3 and week 4, when the plant grew from 40 centimeters to 80 centimeters, a total of 40 centimeters growth.

Circle Graphs or Pie Charts

A *circle graph,* or *pie chart,* shows the relationship between the whole circle (100%) and the various slices that represent portions of that 100%—the larger the slice, the higher the percentage.

For example:

1. Based on the following circle graph:

    A. If Smithville Community Theater has $1,000 to spend this month, how much is spent on set construction?

    B. What is the ratio of the amount of money spent on advertising to the amount of money spent on set construction?

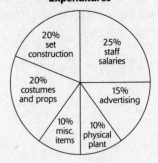

Smithville Community Theater Expenditures

    A. The theater spends 20% of its money on set construction. Twenty percent of $1,000 is $200, so $200 is spent on set construction.

    B. To answer this question, you must use the information in the graph to make a ratio.

$$\frac{\text{advertising}}{\text{set construction}} = \frac{15\% \text{ of } 1000}{20\% \text{ of } 1000} = \frac{150}{200} = \frac{3}{4}$$

Notice that $\frac{15\%}{20\%}$ reduces to $\frac{3}{4}$.

2. Based on the following circle graph:

    A. If the Bell Canyon PTA spends the same percentage on dances every year, how much do they spend on dances in a year in which the total amount spent is $15,000?

    B. The amount of money spent on field trips in 1995 was approximately what percent of the total amount spent?

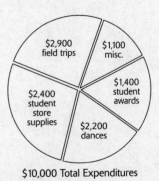

$10,000 Total Expenditures

A. To answer this question, you must find a percent, and then apply this percent to a new total. In 1995, the PTA spent $2,200 on dances. This can be calculated as 22% of the total spent in 1995 by the following method:

$$\frac{2,200}{10,000} = \frac{22}{100} = 22\%$$

Multiplying 22% by the *new* total amount spent ($15,000) gives the right answer.

$$22\% = .22$$
$$.22 \times 15,000 = 3,300 \text{ or } \$3,300$$

You could use another common-sense method. If $2,200 out of $10,000 is spent for dances, $1,100 out of every $5,000 is spent for dances. Since $15,000 is $3 \times \$5,000$, $3 \times \$1,100$ is $3,300.

B. By carefully reading the information in the graph, you find that $2,900 was spent on field trips. The information describing the graph explains that the total expenditures were $10,000. Because $2,900 is approximately $3,000, the approximate percentage is worked out as follows:

$$\frac{3,000}{10,000} = \frac{30}{100} = 30\%$$

Algebra

Algebra Diagnostic Test

Questions

1. The sum of a number and 9 can be written:

2. Evaluate: $3x^2 + 5y + 7$ if $x = -2$ and $y = 3$.

3. Solve for x: $x + 5 = 17$.

4. Solve for x: $4x + 9 = 21$.

5. Solve for x: $5x + 7 = 3x - 9$.

6. Solve for x: $|x| - 4 = 8$.

7. Solve for x: $mx - n = y$.

8. Solve for x: $\frac{r}{x} = \frac{s}{t}$.

9. Solve for y: $\frac{3}{7} = \frac{y}{8}$.

10. Simplify $8xy^2 + 3xy + 4xy^2 - 2xy$.

11. Simplify $6x^2(4x^3y)$.

12. $x^{-5} =$

13. Simplify $(5x + 2z) + (3x - 4z)$.

14. Simplify $(4x - 7z) - (3x - 4z)$.

15. Factor $ab + ac$.

16. Factor $x^2 - 5x - 14$.

17. Solve $x^2 + 7x = -10$.

18. Solve for x: $2x + 3 \leq 11$.

19. Solve for x: $3x + 4 \geq 5x - 8$.

20. Solve for x: $|x - 3| < 6$.

21. Solve for x: $2|x| + 4 \geq 8$.

22. Solve this system for x and y:

$$8x + 2y = 7$$
$$3x - 4y = 5$$

23. Graph $x + y = 6$ on the following graph:

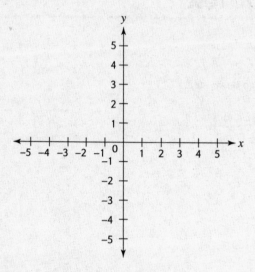

24. What is the slope and the y-intercept of the equation $y = 6x + 2$?

25. What is the equation of the line passing through the points (3,6) and (2,–3)?

Answers

1. $n + 9$ or $9 + n$

2. 34

3. $x = 12$

4. $x = 3$

5. $x = -8$

6. $x = 12$ or -12

7. $x = \dfrac{(y + n)}{m}$

8. $x = \dfrac{rt}{s}$

9. $y = \dfrac{24}{7}$ or $3\dfrac{3}{7}$

10. $12xy^2 + xy$

11. $24x^5y$

12. $\dfrac{1}{x^5}$

13. $8x - 2z$

14. $x - 3z$

15. $a(b + c)$

16. $(x - 7)(x + 2)$

17. $x = -2$ or $x = -5$

18. $x \leq 4$

19. $x \leq 6$

20. $-3 < x < 9$ could also be written $x > -3$ and $x < 9$

21. $x \geq 2$ or $x \leq -2$

22. $x = 1$, $y = -\dfrac{1}{2}$

23.

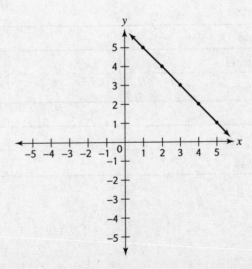

24. Slope = 6, y-intercept = 2

25. $y = 9x - 21$

Algebra Review

Variables and Algebraic Expressions

A *variable* is a symbol used to denote any element of a given set—often a letter used to stand for a number. Variables are used to change verbal expressions into *algebraic expressions*. For example:

Give the algebraic expression:

Verbal Expression	Algebraic Expression
(a) the sum of a number and 7	$n + 7$ or $7 + n$
(b) the number diminished by 10	$n - 10$
(c) seven times a number	$7n$
(d) x divided by 4	$x/4$
(e) five more than the product of 2 and n	$2n + 5$ or $5 + 2n$

These words can be helpful in making algebraic expressions.

Key Words Denoting Addition		
sum	larger than	enlarge
plus	gain	rise
more than	increase	grow
greater than		

Key Words Denoting Subtraction		
difference	smaller than	lower
minus	fewer than	diminish
lose	decrease	reduced
less than	drop	

Key Words Denoting Multiplication		
product	times	of
multiplied by	twice	

Key Words Denoting Division	
quotient	ratio
divided by	half

Evaluating Expressions

To *evaluate* an expression, insert the value for the unknowns and do the arithmetic.

For example:

Evaluate each of the following.

1. $ab + c$ if $a = 5$, $b = 4$ and $c = 3$

$$5(4) + 3 =$$
$$20 + 3 = 23$$

2. $2x^2 + 3y + 6$ if $x = 2$ and $y = 9$

$$2(2^2) + 3(9) + 6 =$$
$$2(4) + 27 + 6 =$$
$$8 + 27 + 6 = 41$$

3. If $x = -4$, then $|6 - x| - |x - 2| =$

$$|6 - (-4)| - |(-4) - 2| =$$
$$|6 + 4| - |-4 - 2| =$$
$$|10| - |-6| =$$
$$10 - 6 = 4$$

Equations

An *equation* is a relationship between numbers and/or symbols. It helps to remember that an equation is like a balance scale, with the equal sign (=) being the fulcrum, or center. Thus, if you do the *same thing to both sides* of the equal sign (say, add 5 to each side), the equation is still balanced. To solve an equation, first you must get the variable you are looking for on one side of the equal sign and everything else on the other side.

For example:

1. Solve for x: $x - 5 = 23$

To solve the equation $x - 5 = 23$, get x by itself on one side; therefore, add 5 to both sides:

$$
\begin{array}{r}
x - 5 = 23 \\
\underline{+5 \quad +5} \\
x \quad\ = 28
\end{array}
$$

In the same manner, subtract, multiply, or divide *both* sides of an equation by the same (nonzero) number, and the equation does not change. Sometimes you have to use more than one step to solve for an unknown.

For example:

2. Solve for x: $3x + 4 = 19$

Subtract 4 from both sides to get the $3x$ by itself on one side:

$$\begin{array}{r} 3x + 4 = 19 \\ \underline{-4 \quad -4} \\ 3x \quad = 15 \end{array}$$

Then divide both sides by 3 to get x:

$$\frac{3x}{3} = \frac{15}{3}$$
$$x = 5$$

3. Solve for x: $6x + 3 = 4x + 5$

Add -3 to each side:

$$\begin{array}{r} 6x + 3 = 4x + 5 \\ \underline{-3 \qquad -3} \\ 6x \quad = 4x + 2 \end{array}$$

Add $-4x$ to each side:

$$\begin{array}{r} 6x = 4x + 2 \\ \underline{-4x \ -4x} \\ 2x = \qquad 2 \end{array}$$

Divide each side by 2:

$$\frac{2x}{2} = \frac{2}{2}$$
$$x = 1$$

Remember: Solving an equation requires using opposite operations until the variable is on one side by itself (for addition, subtract; for multiplication, divide; and so on).

Solving Equations Containing Absolute Value

To solve an equation containing absolute value, isolate the absolute value on one side of the equation. Then, set its contents equal to both + and – the other side of the equation and solve both equations.

For example:

1. Solve for x: $|x| + 2 = 5$

Isolate the absolute value

$$\begin{array}{r} |x| + 2 = \ 5 \\ \underline{-2 \ -2} \\ |x| \quad = \ 3 \end{array}$$

Set the contents of the absolute value portion equal to +3 and –3.

$$x = 3$$
$$x = -3$$

Answer: 3, –3

2. Solve for x: $3|x-1|-1=11$

Isolate the absolute value.

$$3|x-1|-1=11$$
$$\underline{\qquad +1 \quad +1}$$
$$3|x-1| \qquad = 12$$

Divide by 3.

$$\frac{3|x-1|}{3} = \frac{12}{3}$$
$$|x-1| \qquad = 4$$

Set the contents of the absolute value portion equal to +4 and –4.

Solving for x,

$$x-1=4 \qquad x-1=-4$$
$$\underline{+1 \quad +1} \qquad \underline{+1 \quad +1}$$
$$x \quad = 5 \qquad x \quad = -3$$

Answer: 5, –3

Understood Multiplying

When two or more variables, or a number and variables, are written next to each other, they are understood to be multiplied. Thus, $8x$ means 8 times x, ab means a times b, and $18ab$ means 18 times a times b.

Parentheses also represent multiplication. Thus, $(a)b$ means a times b. A raised dot also means multiplication. Thus, $6 \cdot 5$ means 6 times 5.

Literal Equations

Literal equations have no numbers, only symbols (variables). For example:

Solve for Q: $QP - X = Y$

First add X to both sides:

$$QP - X = Y$$
$$\underline{+X \qquad +X}$$
$$QP \qquad = Y+X$$

Then divide both sides by P:

$$\frac{QP}{P} = \frac{Y+X}{P}$$
$$Q = \frac{Y+X}{P}$$

Again opposite operations were used to isolate Q.

Cross Multiplying

Solve for x: $\dfrac{b}{x} = \dfrac{p}{q}$

To solve this equation quickly, cross multiply. To cross multiply:

1. Bring the denominators up next to the numerators on the opposite side.
2. Multiply.

$$\frac{b}{x} = \frac{p}{q}$$

$$bq = px$$

Then, divide both sides by p to get x alone:

$$\frac{bq}{p} = \frac{px}{p}$$

$$\frac{bq}{p} = x \text{ or } x = \frac{bq}{p}$$

Cross multiplying can be used only when the format is two fractions separated by an equal sign.

Proportions

Proportions are written as two fractions equal to each other.

Solve this proportion for x: $\frac{p}{q} = \frac{x}{y}$

This is read "p is to q as x is to y." Cross multiply and solve:

$$py = xq$$

$$\frac{py}{q} = \frac{xq}{q}$$

$$\frac{py}{q} = x \text{ or } x = \frac{py}{q}$$

Monomials and Polynomials

A *monomial* is an algebraic expression that consists of only one term. For instance, $9x$, $4a^2$, and $3mpxz^2$ are all monomials.

A *polynomial* consists of two or more terms; $x + y$, $y^2 - x^2$, and $x^2 + 3x + 5y^2$ are all polynomials.

Adding and Subtracting Monomials

To add or subtract monomials, follow the same rules as with regular signed numbers, provided that the terms are alike:

$$\begin{array}{r} 15x^2yz \\ -18x^2yz \\ \hline -3x^2yz \end{array} \qquad 3x + 2x = 5x$$

Multiplying and Dividing Monomials

To multiply monomials, add the exponents of the same terms:

$$(x^3)(x^4) = x^7$$

$$(x \times x \times x)(x \times x \times x \times x) = x^7$$

To divide monomials, subtract the exponents of like terms:

$$\frac{y^{15}}{y^4} = y^{11} \qquad \frac{x^5 y^2}{x^3 y} = x^2 y \qquad \frac{36a^4 b^6}{-9ab} = -4a^3 b^5$$

Remember: x is the same as x^1.

Working with Negative Exponents

If an exponent is negative, such as x^{-3}, then the variable and exponent can be dropped under the number 1 in a fraction to remove the negative sign, as follows.

$$x^{-3} = \frac{1}{x^3}$$

Another example:

$$a^{-5} = \frac{1}{a^5}$$

A few examples including some with multiplication and division follow:

1. $a^{-2}b = \dfrac{b}{a^2}$

2. $\dfrac{a^{-3}}{b^4} = \dfrac{1}{a^3 b^4}$

3. $\left(a^2 b^{-3}\right)\left(a^{-1} b^4\right) = ab$

   $\begin{bmatrix} a^2 \cdot a^{-1} = a \\ b^{-3} \cdot b^4 = b \end{bmatrix}$

If negative exponent belongs to a number or variable below the fraction bar, then simply bring the number or variable up and drop the negative sign.

4. $\dfrac{1}{x^{-2}} = x^2$

5. $\dfrac{x^6}{x^{-3}} = x^6 \cdot x^3 = x^9$

6. $\left(3x^{-2}\right)^{-2} = 3^{-2} \cdot x^{-2 \cdot -2} = 3^{-2} \cdot x^4 = \dfrac{1}{9} \cdot x^4 = \dfrac{x^4}{9}$

7. $\left(\dfrac{1}{3}\right)^{-2} = \dfrac{1}{\left(\dfrac{1}{3}\right)^2} = \dfrac{1}{\dfrac{1}{9}} = \dfrac{9}{1} = 9$

Or simply invert the fraction and drop the negative sign:

$$\left(\frac{1}{3}\right)^{-2} = \left(\frac{3}{1}\right)^2 = 9$$

If the exponent is a fraction, then the number above the bar is the power, and the number below the bar is the root

For example:

$$3^{\frac{1}{2}} = \sqrt[2]{3^1} = \sqrt{3}$$

(2 is understood in the square root)

A few more examples:

$$5^{\frac{1}{3}} = \sqrt[3]{5^1} = \sqrt[3]{5}$$
$$6^{\frac{2}{3}} = \sqrt[3]{6^2} = \sqrt[3]{36}$$
$$2^{\frac{3}{2}} = \sqrt[2]{2^3} = \sqrt{8} \text{ reduces to } \sqrt{4 \cdot 2} = 2\sqrt{2}$$
$$4^{\frac{1}{4}} = \sqrt[4]{4^1} = \sqrt[4]{4}$$

Adding and Subtracting Polynomials

To add or subtract polynomials, just arrange like terms in columns, and then add or subtract:

Add:

$$
\begin{array}{r}
a^2 + ab + b^2 \\
3a^2 + 4ab - 2b^2 \\
\hline
4a^2 + 5ab - b^2
\end{array}
$$

Subtract:

$$
\begin{array}{r}
a^2 + b^2 \\
(-)\,2a^2 - b^2 \\
\hline
\end{array}
\quad \rightarrow \quad
\begin{array}{r}
a^2 + b^2 \\
+ -2a^2 + b^2 \\
\hline
-a^2 + 2b^2
\end{array}
$$

Multiplying Polynomials

To multiply polynomials, multiply each term in one polynomial by each term in the other polynomials. Then simplify if necessary:

$$(3x + a)(2x - 2a) =$$

$$
\begin{array}{r}
2x - 2a \\
\times\ 3x + a \\
\hline
+2ax - 2a^2 \\
6x^2 - 6ax \\
\hline
6x^2 - 4ax - 2a^2
\end{array}
\qquad \text{similar to} \qquad
\begin{array}{r}
23 \\
\times 19 \\
\hline
207 \\
230 \\
\hline
427
\end{array}
$$

Factoring

To *factor* means to find two or more quantities whose product equals the original quantity.

Factoring Out a Common Factor

Factor $2y^3 - 6y$.

1. Find the largest common monomial factor of each term.
2. Divide the original polynomial by this factor to obtain the second factor. (The second factor is a polynomial.)

$$2y^3 - 6y = 2y(y^2 - 3)$$

Another example: $x^5 - 4x^3 + x^2 = x^2(x^3 - 4x + 1)$

Factoring the Difference Between Two Squares

Factor $x^2 - 144$.

1. Find the square root of the first term and the square root of the second term.
2. Express your answer as the product of the sum of the quantities from step 1 times the difference of those quantities.

$$x^2 - 144 = (x + 12)(x - 12)$$

Another example: $a^2 - b^2 = (a + b)(a - b)$

Another example: $9x^2 - 16y^2 = (3x + 4y)(3x - 4y)$

Note: $x^2 + 144$ is not factorable.

Factoring Polynomials That Have Three Terms: $Ax^2 + Bx + C$

To factor polynomials that have three terms, of the form $Ax^2 + Bx + C$:

1. Check to see if you can monomial factor (factor out common terms). Then, if $A = 1$ (that is, the first term is simply x^2), use double parentheses and factor the first term. Place these factors in the left sides of the parentheses. For example, $(x \quad)(x \quad)$.

2. Factor the last term, and place the factors in the right sides of the parentheses.

To decide on the signs of the numbers, do the following:

If the sign of the last term is *negative*:

1. Find two numbers whose product is the last term and whose *difference* is the *coefficient* (number in front) of the middle term.

2. Give the larger of these two numbers the sign of the middle term, and give the *opposite* sign to the other factor.

If the sign of the last term is *positive*:

1. Find two numbers whose product is the last term and whose sum is the coefficient of the middle term.

2. Give both factors the sign of the middle term.

For example:

1. Factor $x^2 - 3x - 10$.

   First check to see if you can *monomial factor* (factor out common terms). Because this is not possible, use double parentheses and factor the first terms as follows: $(x \quad)(x \quad)$.

   Next, factor the last term (10) into 2 times 5. (Using the preceding information, 5 must take the negative sign and 2 must take the positive sign because they then total the coefficient of the middle term, which is −3.) Add the proper signs, leaving:

   $$(x - 5)(x + 2)$$

   Multiply the means (inner terms) and extremes (outer terms) to check your work.

   $$(x - 5)(x + 2)$$
   $$-5x$$
   $$+2x$$
   $$-3x \text{ (which is the middle term)}$$

   To completely check, multiply the factors together.

   $$\begin{array}{r} x - 5 \\ \times\ x + 2 \\ \hline +2x - 10 \\ x^2 - 5x \\ \hline x^2 - 3x - 10 \end{array}$$

2. Factor $x^2 + 8x + 15$.

   $(x + 3)(x + 5)$

   Notice that $3 \times 5 = 15$ and $3 + 5 = 8$, the coefficient of the middle term. Also, the signs of both factors are +, the sign of the middle term. To check your work:

$$(x + 3)(x + 5)$$
$$+ 3x$$
$$+ 5x$$
$$+ 8x \text{ (the middle term)}$$

If, however, $A \neq 1$ (that is, the first term has a coefficient—for example, $4x^2 + 5x + 1$), then additional trial and error is necessary.

3. Factor $4x^2 + 5x + 1$.

   $(2x + \quad)(2x + \quad)$ might work for the first term. But when 1's are used as factors to get the last term— $(2x + 1)(2x + 1)$—the middle term comes out as $4x$ instead of $5x$.

$$(2x + 1)(2x + 1)$$
$$+ 2x$$
$$+ 2x$$
$$+ 4x$$

   Therefore, try $(4x + \quad)(x + \quad)$. This time, using 1's as factors to get the last terms gives $(4x + 1)(x + 1)$. Checking for the middle term:

$$(4x + 1)(x + 1)$$
$$+ 1x$$
$$+ 4x$$
$$+ 5x$$

   Therefore, $4x^2 + 5x + 1 = (4x + 1)(x + 1)$.

4. Factor $5x^3 + 6x^2 + x$.

   Factoring out an x leaves $x(5x^2 + 6x + 1)$.

   Now, factor as usual giving $x(5x + 1)(x + 1)$.

   To check your work:

$$(5x + 1)(x + 1)$$
$$+ 1x \qquad \text{(the middle term}$$
$$\qquad\qquad \text{after } x \text{ was}$$
$$+ 5x \qquad \text{factored out)}$$
$$+ 6x$$

Solving Quadratic Equations

A *quadratic equation* is an equation that could be written in the form $Ax^2 + Bx + C = 0$. To solve a quadratic equation:

1. Put all terms on one side of the equal sign, leaving zero on the other side.
2. Factor.
3. Set each factor equal to zero.
4. Solve each of these equations.
5. Check by inserting your answer in the original equation.

For example:

1. Solve $x^2 - 6x = 16$.

Following the steps, $x^2 - 6x = 16$ becomes $x^2 - 6x - 16 = 0$.

Factoring, $(x - 8)(x + 2) = 0$

$$x - 8 = 0 \quad \text{or} \quad x + 2 = 0$$
$$x \quad = 8 \qquad x \qquad = -2$$

To check:

$$8^2 - 6(8) = 16 \quad \text{or} \quad (-2)^2 - 6(-2) = 16$$
$$64 - 48 = 16 \quad \text{or} \qquad 4 + 12 = 16$$
$$16 = 16 \quad \text{or} \qquad 16 = 16$$

Both values 8 and −2 are solutions to the original equation.

2. Solve $y^2 = -6y - 5$.

Setting all terms equal to zero:

$$y^2 + 6y + 5 = 0$$

Factoring, $(y + 5)(y + 1) = 0$

Setting each factor to 0:

$$y + 5 = 0 \quad \text{or} \quad y + 1 = 0$$
$$y = -5 \quad \text{or} \qquad y = -1$$

To check:

$$(-5)^2 = -6(-5) - 5 \quad \text{or} \quad (-1)^2 = -6(-1) - 5$$
$$25 = 30 - 5 \quad \text{or} \qquad 1 = 6 - 5$$
$$25 = 25 \quad \text{or} \qquad 1 = 1$$

A quadratic equation with a term missing is called an *incomplete quadratic equation*.

3. Solve $x^2 - 16 = 0$.

Factoring, $(x + 4)(x - 4) = 0$:

$$x + 4 = 0 \quad \text{or} \quad x - 4 = 0$$
$$x = -4 \quad \text{or} \qquad x = 4$$

To check:

$$(-4)^2 - 16 = 0 \quad \text{or} \quad (4)^2 - 16 = 0$$
$$16 - 16 = 0 \quad \text{or} \qquad 16 - 16 = 0$$
$$0 = 0 \quad \text{or} \qquad 0 = 0$$

4. Solve $x^2 + 6x = 0$.

Factoring, $x(x + 6) = 0$:

$$x = 0 \quad \text{or} \quad x + 6 = 0$$
$$x = 0 \quad \text{or} \qquad x = -6$$

To check:

$$(0)^2 + 6(0) = 0 \quad \text{or} \quad (-6)^2 + 6(-6) = 0$$
$$0 + 0 = 0 \quad \text{or} \quad 36 + -36 = 0$$
$$0 = 0 \quad \text{or} \quad 0 = 0$$

Algebraic fractions are fractions using a variable in the numerator or denominator, such as $\frac{3}{x}$. Since division by 0 is impossible, variables in the denominator have certain restrictions. The denominator can never equal 0. Therefore in the fractions

$$\frac{5}{x} \quad x \text{ cannot equal } 0 \ (x \neq 0)$$

$$\frac{2}{x-3} \quad x \text{ cannot equal } 3 \ (x \neq 3)$$

$$\frac{3}{a-b} \quad a - b \text{ cannot equal } 0 \ (a - b \neq 0)$$
$$\text{so } a \text{ cannot equal } b \ (a \neq b)$$

$$\frac{4}{a^2 b} \quad a \text{ cannot equal } 0 \text{ and } b \text{ cannot equal } 0$$
$$(a \neq 0 \text{ and } b \neq 0)$$

Be aware of these types of restrictions.

Operations with Algebraic Fractions

Reducing Algebraic Fractions

To *reduce an algebraic fraction* to lowest terms, first factor the numerator and the denominator; then cancel (or divide out) common factors. For example:

1. Reduce $\dfrac{4x^3}{8x^2}$

$$\frac{\overset{1}{\cancel{4}}\overset{x^1}{\cancel{x^3}}}{\underset{2}{\cancel{8}}\cancel{x^2}} = \frac{1}{2}x$$

2. Reduce $\dfrac{3x-3}{4x-4}$

$$\frac{3x-3}{4x-4} = \frac{3(x-1)}{4(x-1)} = \frac{3\cancel{(x-1)}}{4\cancel{(x-1)}} = \frac{3}{4}$$

3. Reduce $\dfrac{x^2+2x+1}{3x+3}$

$$\frac{x^2+2x+1}{3x+3} = \frac{(x+1)(x+1)}{3(x+1)} = \frac{(x+1)(x+1)}{3\cancel{(x+1)}}$$
$$= \frac{x+1}{3}$$

4. Reduce $\dfrac{x^2-y^2}{x^3-y^3}$

$$\frac{x^2-y^2}{x^3-y^3}=\frac{(x-y)(x+y)}{(x-y)(x^2+xy+y^2)}=$$

$$\frac{\cancel{(x-y)}(x+y)}{\cancel{(x-y)}(x^2+xy+y^2)}=\frac{x+y}{x^2+xy+y^2}$$

Warning: Do *not* cancel through an addition or subtraction sign. For example:

$$\frac{x+1}{x+2}\neq\frac{\cancel{x}+1}{\cancel{x}+2}\neq\frac{1}{2}$$

or

$$\frac{x+6}{6}\neq\frac{x+\cancel{6}}{\cancel{6}}\neq x$$

Multiplying Algebraic Fractions

To *multiply algebraic functions,* first factor the numerator and denominators that are polynomials; then cancel where possible. Multiply the remaining numerators together and denominators together. (If you've canceled properly, your answer will be in reduced form.) For example:

1. $\dfrac{2x}{3}\cdot\dfrac{y}{5}=\dfrac{2x}{3}\cdot\dfrac{y}{5}=\dfrac{2xy}{15}$

2. $\dfrac{x^2}{3y}\cdot\dfrac{2y}{3x}=\dfrac{x^{\cancel{2}}}{3\cancel{y}}\cdot\dfrac{2\cancel{y}}{3\cancel{x}}=\dfrac{2x}{9}$

3. $\dfrac{x+1}{5y+10}\cdot\dfrac{y+2}{x^2+2x+1}=\dfrac{x+1}{5(y+2)}\cdot\dfrac{y+2}{(x+1)(x+1)}=$

$$\frac{\cancel{x+1}}{5\cancel{(y+2)}}\cdot\frac{\cancel{y+2}}{\cancel{(x+1)}(x+1)}=\frac{1}{5(x+1)}$$

Dividing Algebraic Fractions

To *divide algebraic fractions,* invert the fraction following the division sign and multiply. Remember you can cancel only after you invert. For example:

1. $\dfrac{3x^2}{5}\div\dfrac{2x}{y}=\dfrac{3x^2}{5}\cdot\dfrac{y}{2x}=\dfrac{3x^{\cancel{2}^1}}{5}\cdot\dfrac{y}{2\cancel{x}}=\dfrac{3xy}{10}$

2. $\dfrac{4x-8}{6}\div\dfrac{x-2}{3}=\dfrac{4x-8}{6}\cdot\dfrac{3}{x-2}=\dfrac{4(x-2)}{6}\cdot\dfrac{3}{x-2}=$

$$\frac{4\cancel{(x-2)}^1}{{}_2\cancel{6}}\cdot\frac{\cancel{3}^1}{{}_1\cancel{x-2}}=\frac{4}{2}=2$$

Adding or Subtracting Algebraic Fractions

To *add or subtract algebraic fractions having a common denominator,* simply keep the denominator and combine (add or subtract) the numerators. Reduce if necessary. For example:

1. $\dfrac{4}{x} + \dfrac{5}{x} = \dfrac{4+5}{x} = \dfrac{9}{x}$

2. $\dfrac{x-4}{x+1} + \dfrac{3}{x+1} = \dfrac{x-4+3}{x+1} = \dfrac{x-1}{x+1}$

3. $\dfrac{3x}{y} - \dfrac{2x-1}{y} = \dfrac{3x-(2x-1)}{y} = \dfrac{3x-2x+1}{y} = \dfrac{x+1}{y}$

To *add or subtract algebraic fractions having different denominators,* first find a lowest common denominator (LCD), change each fraction to an equivalent fraction with the common denominator, then combine each numerator. Reduce if necessary. For example:

1. $\dfrac{2}{x} + \dfrac{3}{y} =$

   LCD = xy

   $\dfrac{2}{x} \cdot \dfrac{y}{y} + \dfrac{3}{y} \cdot \dfrac{x}{x} = \dfrac{2y}{xy} \cdot \dfrac{3x}{xy} = \dfrac{2y+3x}{xy}$

2. $\dfrac{x+2}{3x} + \dfrac{x-3}{6x} =$

   LCD = $6x$

   $\dfrac{x+2}{3x} \cdot \dfrac{2}{2} + \dfrac{x-3}{6x} = \dfrac{2x+4}{6x} + \dfrac{x-3}{6x} = \dfrac{2x+4+x-3}{6x} = \dfrac{3x+1}{6x}$

If there is a common variable factor with more than one exponent, use its greatest exponent.

3. $\dfrac{2}{y^2} - \dfrac{3}{y} =$

   LCD = y^2

   $\dfrac{2}{y^2} - \dfrac{3}{y} \cdot \dfrac{y}{y} = \dfrac{2}{y^2} - \dfrac{3y}{y^2} = \dfrac{2-3y}{y^2}$

4. $\dfrac{4}{x^3 y} + \dfrac{3}{xy^2} =$

   LCD = $x^3 y^2$

   $\dfrac{4}{x^3 y} \cdot \dfrac{y}{y} + \dfrac{3}{xy^2} \cdot \dfrac{x^2}{x^2} = \dfrac{4y}{x^3 y^2} + \dfrac{3x^2}{x^3 y^2} = \dfrac{4y+3x^2}{x^3 y^2}$

To find *the lowest common denominator,* it is often necessary to factor the denominators and proceed as follows.

$$\frac{x}{3x+3} + \frac{2x}{x+1} = \frac{x}{3(x+1)} + \frac{2x}{x+1}$$

$$\text{LCD} = 3(x+1)$$

$$\frac{x}{3(x+1)} + \frac{2x}{x+1} \cdot \frac{3}{3} = \frac{x}{3(x+1)} + \frac{6x}{3(x+1)} =$$

$$\frac{x+6x}{3(x+1)} = \frac{7x}{3(x+1)}$$

Inequalities

An *inequality* is a statement in which the relationships are not equal. Instead of using an equal sign (=), as in an equation, we use > (greater than) and < (less than), or ≥ (greater than or equal to) and ≤ (less than or equal to).

When working with inequalities, treat them exactly like equations, *except*, when you multiply or divide both sides by a negative number, *reverse* the direction of the sign. For example:

1. Solve for x: $2x + 4 > 6$.

$$2x + 4 > 6$$
$$\underline{-4 \quad -4}$$
$$2x \quad > 2$$
$$\frac{2x}{2} \quad > \frac{2}{2}$$
$$x \quad > 1$$

2. Solve for x: $-7x > 14$.

   Divide by -7 and reverse the sign.

$$\frac{-7x}{-7} < \frac{14}{-7}$$
$$x < -2$$

3. Solve for x: $3x + 2 \geq 5x - 10$.

$$3x + 2 \geq 5x - 10$$
$$\underline{-2 \qquad -2}$$
$$3x \geq 5x - 12$$
$$\underline{-5x \quad -5x}$$
$$-2x \geq \quad -12$$

   Divide both sides by -2 and reverse the sign.

$$\frac{-2x}{-2} \leq \frac{-12}{-2}$$
$$x \leq 6$$

Graphing Inequalities

Examples:

When graphing inequalities involving only integers, dots are used.

1. Graph the set of x such that $1 \leq x \leq 4$ and x is an integer.

   {x: $1 \leq x \leq 4$, x is an integer}

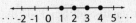

When graphing inequalities involving real numbers; lines, rays, and dots are used. A *dot* is used if the number is included. A *hollow dot* is used if the number is not included.

2. Graph the set of x such that $x \geq 1$.   {x: $x \geq 1$}

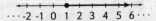

3. Graph the set of x such that $x > 1$. $\{x : x > 1\}$

$$\cdots \text{-3 -2 -1 0 1 2 3 4} \cdots$$

4. Graph the set of x such that $x < 4$. $\{x : x < 4\}$

$$\cdots \text{-3 -2 -1 0 1 2 3 4} \cdots$$

This ray is often called an *open ray* or *half line*. The hollow dot distinguishes an open ray from a ray.

Solving Inequalities Containing Absolute Value

To solve an inequality containing absolute value, follow the same steps as solving equations with absolute value, except *reverse* the direction of the sign when setting the absolute value opposite a negative.

For example:

1. Solve for x: $|x - 1| > 2$.

Isolate the absolute value.

$$|x - 1| > 2$$

Set the contents of the absolute value portion to both 2 and –2. Be sure to change the direction of the sign when using –2.

Solve for x.

$$
\begin{array}{ccc}
x - 1 > 2 & & x - 1 < -2 \\
\underline{+1 \ +1} & \text{or} & \underline{+1 \ \ +1} \\
x \quad > 3 & & x \quad < -1
\end{array}
$$

Graph answer:

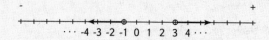

$$- \qquad\qquad\qquad\qquad\qquad\qquad +$$
$$\cdots \text{-4 -3 -2 -1 0 1 2 3 4} \cdots$$

2. Solve for x: $3|x| - 2 \leq 1$.

Isolate the absolute value.

$$
\begin{array}{rl}
3|x| - 2 \leq & 1 \\
\underline{+2 \ +2} & \\
3|x| \leq & 3 \\
\dfrac{3|x|}{3} \leq & \dfrac{3}{3} \\
|x| \leq & 1
\end{array}
$$

Set the contents of the absolute value portion to both 1 and –1. Be sure to change the direction of the sign when using –1.

$$x \leq 1 \text{ and } x \geq -1$$

Graph answer:

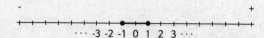

$$- \qquad\qquad\qquad\qquad\qquad\qquad +$$
$$\cdots \text{-3 -2 -1 0 1 2 3} \cdots$$

Solving for Two Unknowns—Systems of Equations

If you solve for two equations with the same two unknowns in each one, you can solve for both unknowns. There are three common methods for solving: addition/subtraction, substitution, and graphing.

Addition/Subtraction Method

To use the addition/subtraction method:

1. Multiply one or both equations by some number to make the number in front of one of the variables (the unknowns) the same in each equation.
2. Add or subtract the two equations to eliminate one variable.
3. Solve for the other unknown.
4. Insert the value of the first unknown in one of the original equations to solve for the second unknown.

For example:

1. Solve for x and y:

$$3x + 3y = 24$$
$$2x + y = 13$$

First multiply the bottom equation by 3. Now the y is preceded by a 3 in each equation.

$$3x + 3y = 24 \qquad\qquad 3x + 3y = 24$$
$$3(2x) + 3(y) = 3(13) \qquad\qquad 6x + 3y = 39$$

Now you can subtract equations, eliminating the y terms.

$$
\begin{aligned}
3x + 3y &= 24 \\
-6x + -3y &= -39 \\
\hline
-3x &= -15 \\
\frac{-3x}{-3} &= \frac{-15}{-3} \\
x &= 5
\end{aligned}
$$

Now insert $x = 5$ in one of the original equations to solve for y.

$$
\begin{aligned}
2x + y &= 13 \\
2(5) + y &= 13 \\
10 + y &= 13 \\
-10 \qquad -10 & \\
\hline
y &= 3
\end{aligned}
$$

Answer: $x = 5$, $y = 3$

Of course, if the number in front of a variable is already the same in each equation, you do not have to change either equation. Simply add or subtract.

2. Solve for x and y:

$$x + y = 7$$
$$x - y = 3$$

$$x + y = 7$$
$$\underline{x - y = 3}$$
$$2x = 10$$
$$\frac{2x}{2} = \frac{10}{2}$$
$$x = 5$$

Now, inserting 5 for x in the first equation gives:

$$5 + y = 7$$
$$\underline{-5 -5}$$
$$y = 2$$

Answer: $x = 5$, $y = 2$

You should note that this method does not work when the two equations are, in fact, the same.

3. Solve for a and b:

$$3a + 4b = 2$$
$$6a + 8b = 4$$

The second equation is actually the first equation multiplied by 2. In this instance, the system is unsolvable.

4. Solve for p and q:

$$3p + 4q = 9$$
$$2p + 2q = 6$$

Multiply the second equation by 2.

$$(2)2p + (2)2q = (2)6$$
$$4p + 4q = 12$$

Now subtract the equations.

$$3p + 4q = 9$$
$$\underline{(-)\,4p + 4q = 12}$$
$$-p = -3$$
$$p = 3$$

Now that you know $p = 3$, you can plug in 3 for p in either of the two original equations to find q.

$$3p + 4q = 9$$
$$3(3) + 4q = 9$$
$$9 + 4q = 9$$
$$4q = 0$$
$$q = 0$$

Answer: $p = 3$, $q = 0$

Substitution Method

Sometimes a system is more easily solved by the substitution method. This method involves substituting one equation into another.

For example:

Solve for x and y when $x = y + 8$ and $x + 3y = 48$.

1. From the first equation, substitute $(y + 8)$ for x in the second equation.

$$(y + 8) + 3y = 48$$

2. Now solve for y. Simplify by combining y's.

$$
\begin{aligned}
4y + 8 &= 48 \\
-8 &= -8 \\
\hline
4y &= 40 \\
\frac{4y}{4} &= \frac{40}{4} \\
y\phantom{\frac{4}{4}} &= 10
\end{aligned}
$$

3. Now insert $y = 10$ in one of the original equations.

$$
\begin{aligned}
x &= y + 8 \\
x &= 10 + 8 \\
x &= 18
\end{aligned}
$$

Answer: $y = 10$, $x = 18$

Graphing Method

Another method of solving equations is by graphing each equation on a coordinate graph. The coordinates of the intersection are the solution to the system. If you are unfamiliar with coordinate graphing, carefully review the "Basic Coordinate Geometry" section before attempting this method.

For example, solve the following system by graphing:

$$
\begin{aligned}
x &= 4 + y \\
x - 3y &= 4
\end{aligned}
$$

1. First, find three values for x and y that satisfy each equation. (Although only two points are necessary to determine a straight line, finding a third point is a good way of checking.)

$$x = 4 + y \qquad\qquad x - 3y = 4$$

x	y
4	0
2	-2
5	1

x	y
1	-1
4	0
7	1

2. Now graph the two lines on the coordinate plane, as shown in the following figure.

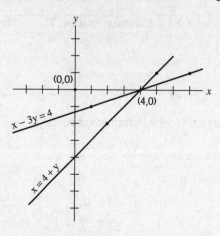

3. The point where the two lines cross (4, 0) is the solution of the system.
4. If the lines are parallel, they do not intersect; there is no solution to the system.

Note: If lines are parallel, they have the same slope.

Basic Coordinate Geometry

Coordinate Graphs (*x-y* Graphs)

A *coordinate graph* is formed by two perpendicular number lines. These lines are called *coordinate axes*. The horizontal axis is called the *x-axis* or the *abscissa*. The vertical line is called the *y-axis* or the *ordinate*. The point at which the two lines intersect is called the *origin* and is represented by the coordinates (0, 0), often marked simply 0.

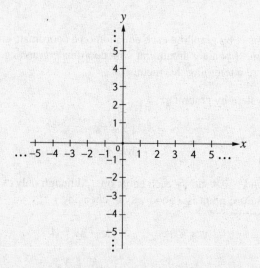

Each point on a coordinate graph is located by an ordered pair of numbers called *coordinates*. Notice the placement of points on the following graph and the coordinates, or ordered pairs, that show their location. Numbers are not usually written on the *x*- and *y*-axes.

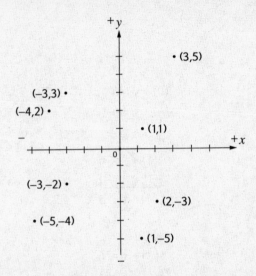

On the *x*-axis, the numbers to the right of 0 are positive and to the left of 0 are negative. On the *y*-axis, numbers above 0 are positive and numbers below 0 are negative. The first number in the ordered pair is called the *x-coordinate* and shows how far to the right or left of 0 the point is. The second number is called the *y-coordinate* and shows how far up or down the point is from 0. The coordinates, or ordered pairs, are shown as (*x, y*). The order of these numbers is very important, as the point (3, 2) is different from the point (2, 3). Also, don't combine the ordered pair of numbers, because they refer to different directions.

The coordinate graph is divided into four quarters called *quadrants*. These quadrants are labeled as follows.

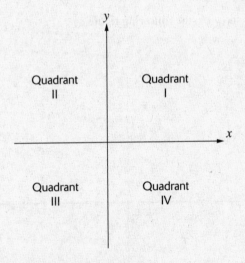

- In Quadrant I, *x* is always positive and *y* is always positive.
- In Quadrant II, *x* is always negative and *y* is always positive.
- In Quadrant III, *x* is always negative and *y* is always negative.
- In Quadrant IV, *x* is always positive and *y* is always negative.

Graphing Equations on the Coordinate Plane

To graph an equation on the coordinate plane, find the solutions by giving a value to one variable and solving the resulting equation for the other variable. Repeat this process to find other solutions. (When giving a value for one variable, start with 0; then try 1, and so forth.) Then, graph the solutions.

For example:

1. Graph the equation $x + y = 6$.

   If x is 0, then y is 6.

$$(0) + y = 6$$
$$y = 6$$

   If x is 1, then y is 5.

$$\begin{aligned} (1) + y &= 6 \\ -1 \quad\quad &-1 \\ \hline y &= 5 \end{aligned}$$

   If x is 2, then y is 4.

$$\begin{aligned} (2) + y &= 6 \\ -2 \quad\quad &-2 \\ \hline y &= 4 \end{aligned}$$

Using a simple chart is helpful.

x	y
0	6
1	5
2	4

Now, plot these coordinates as shown in the following figure.

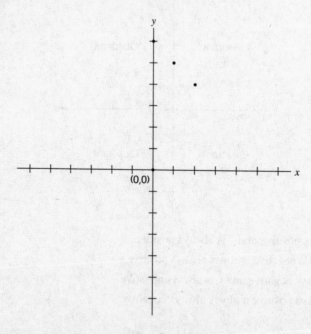

These solutions, when plotted, form a straight line. Equations whose graphs of their solution sets form a straight line are called *linear equations*. Equations that have a variable raised to a power, show division by a variable and involve variables with square roots. Variables multiplied together do not form a straight line when their solutions are graphed. These are called *nonlinear equations*.

2. Graph the equation $y = x^2 + 4$.

If x is 0, then y is 4.

$$y = (0)^2 + 4$$
$$y = 0 + 4$$
$$y = 4$$

If x is 1, then y is 5.

$$y = (1)^2 + 4$$
$$y = 1 + 4$$
$$y = 5$$

If x is 2, then y is 8.

$$y = (2)^2 + 4$$
$$y = 4 + 4$$
$$y = 8$$

Use a simple chart.

x	y
0	4
1	5
2	8

Now, plot these coordinates as shown in the following figure.

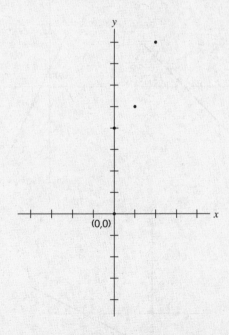

These solutions, when plotted, give a curved line (nonlinear). The more points plotted, the easier it is to see the curve and describe the solution set.

Slope and Intercept of Linear Equations

Two relationships between the graph of a linear equation and the equation itself must be pointed out. One involves the slope of the line, and the other involves the point where the line crosses the y-axis. To see either of these relationships, the terms of the equation must be in a certain order.

$$(+)(1)y = (\ )x + (\ )$$

When the terms are written in this order, the equation is said to be in y-intercept or slope-intercept form. y-form is written $y = mx + b$, and the two relationships involve m and b.

For example:

Write the equations in y-intercept form.

1. $x - y = 3$

    $-y = -x + 3$

    $y = x - 3$

2. $y = -2x + 1$ (already in y-intercept form)

3. $x - 2y = 4$

    $-2y = -x + 4$

    $2y = x - 4$

    $y = \frac{1}{2}x - 2$

As shown in the graphs of the three problems in the following figure, the lines cross the y-axis at -3, $+1$, and -2, the last term in each equation.

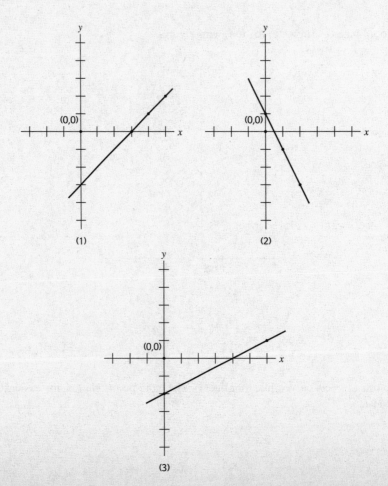

(1)

(2)

(3)

If a linear equation is written in the form $y = mx + b$, b is the y-intercept.

The slope of a line is defined as:

$$\frac{\text{the change in } y}{\text{the change in } x}$$

The word *change* refers to the difference in the value of y (or x) between two points on a line.

$$\text{slope of line } AB = \frac{y_A - y_B}{x_A - x_B} = \frac{y \text{ at point } A - y \text{ at point } B}{x \text{ at point } A - x \text{ at point } B}$$

Note: Points A and B can be any two points on a line; there is no difference in the slope.

1. Find the slope of $x - y = 3$ using coordinates.

   To find the slope of the line, pick any two points on the line, such as A(3, 0) and B (5, 2), and calculate the slope.

   $$\text{slope} = \frac{y_A - y_B}{x_A - x_B} = \frac{(0) - (2)}{(3) - (5)} = \frac{-2}{-2} = 1$$

2. Find the slope of $y = -2x - 1$ using coordinates.

   Pick two points, such as A(1, −3) and B(−1, 1), and calculate the slope.

   $$\text{slope} = \frac{y_A - y_B}{x_A - x_B} = \frac{(-3) - (1)}{(1) - (-1)} = \frac{-3 - 1}{1 + 1} = \frac{-4}{2} = -2$$

Looking back at the equations for examples 1, 2, and 3 written in y-intercept form, it should be evident that the slope of the line is the same as the numerical coefficient of the x term.

1.
   $$y = x - 3$$
   slope $= 1$ y-intercept $= -3$

2.
   $$y = -2x + 1$$
   slope $= -2$ y-intercept $= 1$

3.
   $$y = \tfrac{1}{2}x - 2$$
   slope $= \tfrac{1}{2}$ y-intercept $= -2$

Graphing Linear Equations Using Slope and Intercept

Graphing an equation using its slope and y-intercept is usually quite easy.

1. State the equation in y-intercept form.
2. Locate the y-intercept on the graph (that is, one of the points on the line).
3. Write the slope as a ratio (fraction), and use it to locate other points on the line.
4. Draw a line through the points.

For example:

1. Graph the equation $x - y = 2$ using slope and y-intercept.

   $$x - y = 2$$
   $$-y = -x + 2$$
   $$y = x - 2$$

Locate −2 on the *x*-axis and, from this point, count as shown in the following figure:

slope = 1

or $\dfrac{1}{1}$ $\left(\begin{array}{l}\text{for every 1 up}\\\text{go 1 to the right}\end{array}\right)$

or $\dfrac{-1}{-1}$ $\left(\begin{array}{l}\text{for every 1 down}\\\text{go 1 to the left}\end{array}\right)$

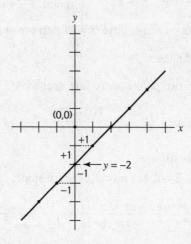

2. Graph the equation $2x - y = -4$ using slope and *y*-intercept.

$$2x - y = -4$$
$$-y = -2x - 4$$
$$y = 2x + 4$$

Locate +4 on the *y*-axis and, from this point, count as shown in the following figure:

slope = 2

or $\dfrac{2}{1}$ $\left(\begin{array}{l}\text{for every 2 up}\\\text{go 1 to the right}\end{array}\right)$

or $\dfrac{-2}{-1}$ $\left(\begin{array}{l}\text{for every 2 down}\\\text{go 1 to the left}\end{array}\right)$

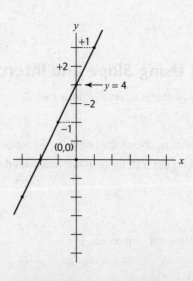

Finding the Equation of a Line

To find the equation of a line when working with ordered pairs, slopes, and intercepts, use the following approach.

1. Find the slope, m.
2. Find the y-intercept, b.
3. Substitute the slope and intercept into the slope-intercept form, $y = mx + b$.
4. Change the slope-intercept form to standard form, $Ax + By = C$.

For example:

1. Find the equation of the line when $m = -4$ and $b = 3$.
   Find the slope, m.

   $$m = -4 \text{ (given)}$$

   Find the y-intercept, b.

   $$b = 3 \text{ (given)}$$

   Substitute the slope and intercept into the slope-intercept form $y = mx + b$.

   $$y = -4x + 3$$

   Change the slope-intercept form to standard form $Ax + By = C$. Since

   $$y = -4x + 3$$

   Adding $4x$ to each side gives:

   $$4x + y = 3$$

2. Find the equation of the line passing through the point (6, 4) with a slope of -3.
   Find the slope, m.

   $$m = -3 \text{ (given)}$$

   Find the y-intercept, b.
   Substitute $m = -3$ and the point (6, 4) into the slope-intercept form to find b.

   $$y = mx + b \text{ where } y = 4, m = -3, \text{ and } x = 6$$
   $$4 = (-3)(6) + b$$
   $$4 = -18 + b$$
   $$18 + 4 = b$$
   $$22 = b$$

   Substitute the slope and intercept into the slope-intercept form: $y = mx + b$.
   Since $m = -3$ and $b = 22$, $y = -3x + 22$.
   Change the slope-intercept form to standard form: $Ax + By = C$.
   Since $y = -3x + 22$, adding $3x$ to each side gives $3x + y = 22$.

3. Find the equation of the line passing through points (5, -4) and (3, -2).
   Find the slope, m.

   $$m = \frac{\text{change in } y}{\text{change in } x} = \frac{(-4)-(-2)}{(5)-(3)} = \frac{-4+2}{2} = \frac{-2}{2} = -1$$

   Find the y-intercept, b.

Substitute the slope and either point into slope-intercept form.

$$y = mx + b \text{ where } m = -1, x = 5, \text{ and } y = -4$$
$$-4 = (-1)(5) + b$$
$$-4 = -5 + b$$
$$5 + -4 = b$$
$$1 = b$$

Substitute the slope and intercept into the slope-intercept form: $y = mx + b$.

Since $m = -1$ and $b = 1$, $y = -1x + 1$ or $y = -x + 1$.

Change the slope-intercept form to standard form: $Ax + By = C$.

Since $y = -x + 1$, adding x to each side gives $x + y = 1$.

Geometry

Geometry Diagnostic Test

Questions

1. Lines that stay the same distance apart and never meet are called _____ lines.

2. Lines that meet to form 90° angles are called _____ lines.

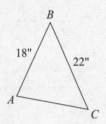

3. In the preceding triangle, *AC* must be smaller than _____ inches.

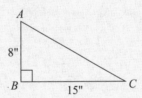

4. What is the length of *AC* in the preceding figure?

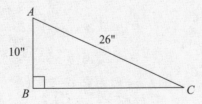

5. What is the length of *BC* in the preceding figure?

6. Name each of the following polygons:

A.

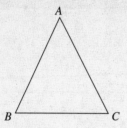

B.

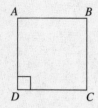

$AB = BC = CD = AD$
$\angle A = \angle B = \angle C = \angle D = 90°$

C.

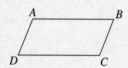

$\overline{AB} \parallel \overline{DC}$
$AB = DC$
$\overline{AD} \parallel \overline{BC}$
$AD = BC$
$\angle A = \angle C$

D.

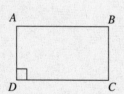

E.

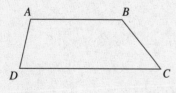

$\overline{AB} \parallel \overline{DC}$

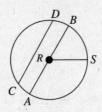

7. Fill in the blanks for circle *R* in the preceding figure:

    A. $\overline{RS}$ is called the _____.

    B. $\overline{AB}$ is called the _____.

    C. $\overline{CD}$ is called a _____.

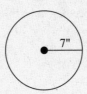

8. Find the area and circumference for the circle in the preceding figure ($\pi \approx \frac{22}{7}$):

    A. area =

    B. circumference =

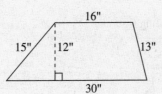

9. Find the area and perimeter of the preceding figure:

    A. area =

    B. perimeter =

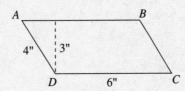

10. Find the area and perimeter of the preceding figure (*ABCD* is a parallelogram):

    A. area =

    B. perimeter =

11. Find the volume of the preceding figure if $V = (\pi r^2)h$. (Use 3.14 for π):

12. What is the surface area and volume of the preceding cube?

    A. surface area =

    B. volume =

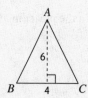

13. What is the area of $\triangle ABC$ in the preceding figure?

Answers

1. parallel

2. perpendicular

3. 40 inches

   (Since $AB + BC = 40$ inches, $AC < AB + BC$ and $AC < 40$ inches.)

4. $AC = 17$ inches

5. Since $\triangle ABC$ is a right triangle, use the Pythagorean theorem:

$$a^2 + b^2 = c^2$$
$$10^2 + b^2 = 26^2$$
$$100 + b^2 = 676$$
$$b^2 = 576$$
$$b = 24"$$

6. A.   triangle
   B.   square
   C.   parallelogram
   D.   rectangle
   E.   trapezoid

7. A.   radius
   B.   diameter
   C.   chord

8. A.   area $= \pi r^2$
   $$= \pi(7^2)$$
   $$= \frac{22}{7}(7)(7)$$
   $$= 154 \text{ square inches}$$
   B.   circumference $= \pi d$
   $$= \pi(14) \ (d = 14", \text{ because } r = 7")$$
   $$= \frac{22}{7}(14)$$
   $$= 22(2)$$
   $$= 44 \text{ inches}$$

9. A.   area $= \frac{1}{2}(a+b)h$
   $$= \frac{1}{2}(16+30)12$$
   $$= \frac{1}{2}(46)12$$
   $$= 23(12)$$
   $$= 276 \text{ square inches}$$
   B.   perimeter $= 16 + 13 + 30 + 15 = 74$ inches

10. A.   area $= bh$
    $$= 6(3)$$
    $$= 18 \text{ square inches}$$
    B.   perimeter $= 6 + 4 + 6 + 4 = 20$ inches

11. volume $= (\pi r^2)h$
$\qquad = (\pi \cdot 10^2)(12)$
$\qquad = 3.14(100)(12)$
$\qquad = 314(12)$
$\qquad = 3{,}768$ cubic inches

12. A. All six surfaces have an area of 4×4, or 16 square inches because each surface is a square. Therefore, 16(6) = 96 square inches is the surface area.

B. Volume $=$ side $\times$ side $\times$ side, or $4^3 = 64$ cubic inches.

13. 12

The area of a triangle is $\frac{1}{2} \times$ base $\times$ height.

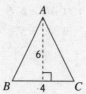

Base AB of the triangle is 4 units (because from A to the y-axis is 2 units and from the y-axis to B is another 2 units). Height BC of the triangle is 6 units (3 units from B to the x-axis and another 3 units to C). Note that $\angle B$ is a right angle.

$$\text{area of triangle} = \frac{1}{2} \times 4 \times 6$$
$$= \frac{1}{2} \times 24$$
$$= 12$$

Geometry Review

Types of Angles

Adjacent angles are any angles that share a common side and a common vertex (point).

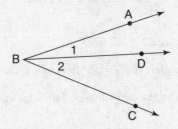

In the diagram, ∠1 and ∠2 are adjacent angles.

A *right angle* has a measure of 90°. The symbol ⌐ in the interior of an angle designates the fact that a right angle is formed.

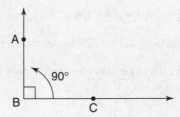

In the diagram, ∠ABC is a right angle.

Any angle that measures less than 90° is called an *acute angle*.

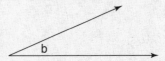

In the diagram, ∠b is acute.

Any angle that measures larger than 90° but smaller than 180° is called an *obtuse angle*.

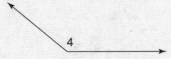

In the diagram, ∠4 is an obtuse angle.

A *straight angle* has a measure of 180°.

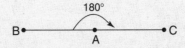

In the diagram, ∠BAC is a straight angle (also called a line).

Two angles whose sum is 90° are called *complementary angles*.

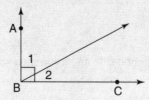

In the diagram, because $\angle ABC$ is a right angle, $\angle 1 + \angle 2 = 90°$.

Therefore, $\angle 1$ and $\angle 2$ are complementary angles. If $\angle 1 = 55°$, its complement, $\angle 2$, would be $90° - 55° = 35°$.

Two angles whose sum is 180° are called *supplementary angles*. Two adjacent angles that form a straight line are supplementary.

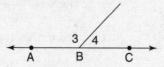

In the diagram, since $\angle ABC$ is a straight angles, $\angle 3 + \angle 4 = 180°$.

Therefore, $\angle 3$ and $\angle 4$ are supplementary angles. If $\angle 3 = 122°$, its supplement, $\angle 4$, would be: $180° - 122° = 58°$.

A ray from the vertex of an angle that divides the angle into two equal pieces is called an *angle bisector*.

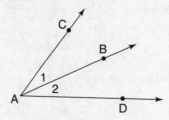

In the diagram, $\overrightarrow{AB}$ is the angle bisector of $\angle CAD$.

Therefore, $\angle 1 = \angle 2$.

If two straight lines intersect, they do so at a point. Four angles are formed. Those angles opposite each other are called *vertical angles*. Those angles sharing a common side and a common vertex are, again, *adjacent angles*. Vertical angles are always equal.

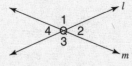

In the diagram, line *l* and line *m* intersect at point *Q*, $\angle 1$, $\angle 2$, $\angle 3$, and $\angle 4$ are formed.

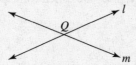

$\left.\begin{array}{l}\angle 1 \text{ and } \angle 3 \\ \angle 2 \text{ and } \angle 4\end{array}\right\}$ are vertical angles

$\left.\begin{array}{l}\angle 1 \text{ and } \angle 2 \\ \angle 2 \text{ and } \angle 3 \\ \angle 3 \text{ and } \angle 4 \\ \angle 1 \text{ and } \angle 4\end{array}\right\}$ are adjacent angles

Therefore, $\begin{array}{l}\angle 1 = \angle 3 \\ \angle 2 = \angle 4\end{array}$

Types of Lines

Two or more lines that cross each other at a point are called *intersecting lines*. That point is on each of those lines.

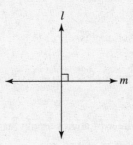

In the diagram, lines *l* and *m* intersect at *Q*.

Two lines that meet to form right angles (90° angles) are called *perpendicular lines*. The symbol ⊥ is used to denote perpendicular lines.

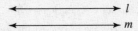

In the diagram, $l \perp m$.

Two or more lines that remain the same distance apart at all times are called *parallel lines*. Parallel lines never meet. The symbol ‖ is used to denote parallel lines.

In the diagram, $l \| m$.

Parallel Lines Cut by Transversal

When two parallel lines are both intersected by the third line, it is termed *parallel lines, cut by a transversal*. In the diagram below, line *n* is the transversal, and lines *m* and *l* are parallel. Eight angles are formed. There are many facts and relationships about these angles.

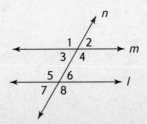

1. *Adjacent angles*. Angles 1 and 2 are adjacent, and they form a straight line; therefore, they are supplementary. $\angle 1 + \angle 2 = 180°$.

   Likewise: $\angle 2 + \angle 4 = 180°$ $\angle 7 + \angle 8 = 180°$

                $\angle 3 + \angle 4 = 180°$ $\angle 5 + \angle 7 = 180°$

                $\angle 1 + \angle 3 = 180°$ $\angle 6 + \angle 8 = 180°$

                $\angle 5 + \angle 6 = 180°$

2. *Vertical angles*. Angles 1 and 4 are vertical angles; therefore, they are equal. $\angle 1 = \angle 4$.

   Likewise: $\angle 2 = \angle 3$

                $\angle 5 = \angle 8$

                $\angle 7 = \angle 6$

3. *Corresponding angles*. If we could physically pick up line *l* and place it on line *m*, the angles that would coincide with each other would be equal in measure. They are called corresponding angles.

   Therefore: $\angle 1 = \angle 5$ $\angle 3 = \angle 7$

               $\angle 2 = \angle 6$ $\angle 4 = \angle 8$

4. *Alternate interior and exterior angles*. Alternate angles are on the opposite side of the transversal. Interior angles are those contained within the parallel lines. Exterior angles are those on the outsides of the parallel lines.

   Therefore: $\angle 3$ and $\angle 6$ are alternate interior angles.

               $\angle 3 = \angle 6$

               $\angle 4$ and $\angle 5$ are alternate interior angles.

               $\angle 4 = \angle 5$

               $\angle 2$ and $\angle 7$ are alternate exterior angles.

               $\angle 2 = \angle 7$

               $\angle 1$ and $\angle 8$ are alternate exterior angles.

               $\angle 1 = \angle 8$

5. *Consecutive interior angles*. Consecutive interior angles are on the same side of the transversal.

   Therefore: $\angle 3$ and $\angle 5$ are consecutive interior angles.

               $\angle 3 = \angle 5 = 180°$

               $\angle 4$ and $\angle 6$ are consecutive interior angles.

               $\angle 4 = \angle 6 = 180°$

The sum of the measures of each pair of consecutive angles $= 180°$.

Using all of these facts, if we are given the measure of one of the eight angles, the other angle measures can all be determined. For example:

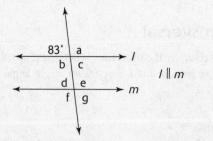

Note that since the lines are parallel, you can *see* which angles are equal, even if you cannot remember the rules.

Polygons

Closed shapes or figures with three or more sides are called *polygons*. (*Poly* means many; *gon* means sides; thus, *polygon* means many sides.)

Triangles

This section deals with those polygons having the fewest number of sides. A *triangle* is a three-sided polygon. It has three angles in its interior. The sum of these angles is *always* 180°. The symbol for triangle is △. A triangle is named by all three letters of its vertices.

The following figure shows △ABC:

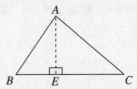

There are various types of triangles:

- A triangle having all three sides equal (meaning all three sides having the same length) is called an *equilateral triangle*.
- A triangle having two sides equal is called an *isosceles triangle*.
- A triangle having none of its sides equal is called a *scalene triangle*.
- A triangle having a right (90°) angle in its interior is called a *right triangle*.

Facts about triangles:

- Every triangle has a base (bottom side) and a height (or altitude). Every height is the *perpendicular* (forming a right angle) distance from a vertex to its opposite side (the base).

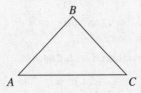

In this diagram of △ABC, $\overline{BC}$ is the base, and $\overline{AE}$ is the height. $\overline{AE} \perp \overline{BC}$.

- The sum of the lengths of any two sides of a triangle must be larger than the length of the third side.
  In the diagram of △ABC:

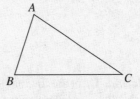

$$AB + BC > AC$$
$$AB + AC > BC$$
$$AC + BC > AB$$

Pythagorean theorem:

- In any right triangle, the relationship between the lengths of the sides is stated by the Pythagorean theorem.

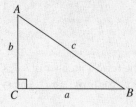

The parts of a right triangle are:

$\angle C$ is the right angle.

- The side opposite the right angle is called the *hypotenuse* (side *c*). (The hypotenuse is always the longest side.) The other two sides are called the *legs* (sides *a* and *b*).

The three lengths *a*, *b*, and *c* are always numbered such that:

$$a^2 + b^2 = c^2$$

For example: If $a = 3$, $b = 4$ and $c = 5$:

$$a^2 + b^2 = c^2$$
$$3^2 + 4^2 = 5^2$$
$$9 + 16 = 25$$
$$25 = 25$$

- Therefore, 3–4–5 is called a Pythagorean triple. There are other values for *a*, *b* and *c* that always work. Some are 1–1–$\sqrt{2}$, 5–12–13, and 8–15–17. Any multiple of one of these triples also works. For example, multiplying the 3–4–5 solution set shows that 6–8–10, 9–12–15, and 15–20–25 are also Pythagorean triples.
- If perfect squares are known, the lengths of these sides can be determined easily. A knowledge of the use of algebraic equations can also be used to determine the lengths of the sides.

For example:

Find the length of *x* in the triangle.

$$a^2 + b^2 = c^2$$
$$x^2 + 10^2 = 15^2$$
$$x^2 + 100 = 225$$
$$x^2 = 125$$
$$x = \sqrt{125}$$
$$\sqrt{125} = \sqrt{25} \times \sqrt{5} = 5\sqrt{5}$$

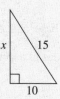

So, $x = 5\sqrt{5}$

Quadrilaterals

A polygon having four sides is called a *quadrilateral*. There are four angles in its interior. The sum of these interior angles is always 360°. A quadrilateral is named using the four letters of its vertices.

The following figure shows quadrilateral *ABCD*.

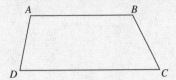

Types of quadrilaterals:

- A *square* has four equal sides and four right angles.

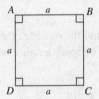

- A *rectangle* has opposite sides that are equal and four right angles.

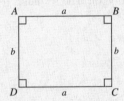

- A *parallelogram* has opposite sides equal and parallel, opposite angles equal, and consecutive angles supplementary. Every parallelogram has a height.

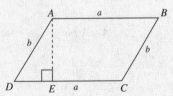

$\overline{AE}$ is the height of the parallelogram, $\overline{AB}\|\overline{CD}$, and $\overline{AD}\|\overline{BC}$.

- A *rhombus* is a parallelogram with four equal sides. A rhombus has a height. $\overline{BE}$ is the height.

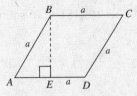

- A *trapezoid* has only one pair of parallel sides. A trapezoid has a height. $\overline{AE}$ is the height. $\overline{AB}\|\overline{DC}$.

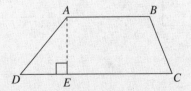

Other Polygons

- A *pentagon* is a 5-sided polygon.
- A *hexagon* is a 6-sided polygon.
- An *octagon* is an 8-sided polygon.
- A *nonagon* is a 9-sided polygon.
- A *decagon* is a 10-sided polygon.

Perimeter

Perimeter means the total distance all the way around the outside of any shape. The perimeter of any polygon can be determined by adding the lengths of all the sides. The total distance around is the sum of all sides of the polygon. No special formulas are really necessary.

Area

Area (A) means the amount of space inside the polygon. The formulas for each area are as follows:

Triangle: $A = \frac{1}{2} bh$

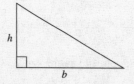 or

For example:

$$A = \frac{1}{2} bh$$

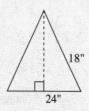

$$A = \frac{1}{2}(24)(18) = 216 \text{ sq in}$$

Square or rectangle: $A = lw$

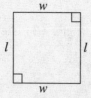 or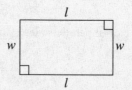

For example:

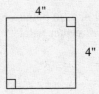

$A = l(w) = 4(4) = 16$ sq in

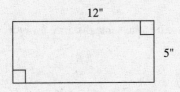

$A = l(w) = 12(5) = 60$ sq in

Parallelogram: $A = bh$

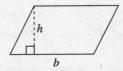

For example:

$A = b(h)$

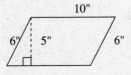

$A = 10(5) = 50$ sq in

Trapezoid: $A = \frac{1}{2}(b_1 + b_2)h$

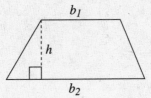

For example:

$A = \frac{1}{2}(b_1 + b_2)h$

$A = \frac{1}{2}(8 + 12)(7)$

$= \frac{1}{2}(20)(7) = 70$ sq in

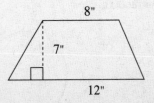

Circles

A closed shape whose side is formed by one curved line, all points on which are equidistant from the center point, is called a *circle*. Circles are named by the letter of their center point.

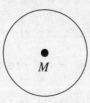

This is circle *M*. *M* is the center point because it is the same distance away from all points on the circle.

Parts of a Circle

■ *Radius* is the distance from a center to any point on a circle. In any circle, all radii (plural) are the same length.

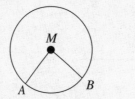

$\overline{MA}$ is a radius.
$\overline{MB}$ is a radius.

■ *Diameter* is the distance across a circle, through the center. In any circle, all diameters are the same length. Each diameter is two radii.

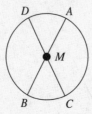

$\overline{AB}$ is a diameter.
$\overline{CD}$ is a diameter.

■ The *chord* is a line segment whose end points lie on the circle itself.

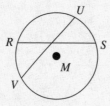

$\overline{RS}$ is a chord.
$\overline{UV}$ is a chord.

The diameter is the longest chord in any circle.

■ An *arc* is the distance between any two points on the circle itself. An arc is a piece of the circle. The symbol ⌒ is used to denote an arc. It is written on top of the two endpoints that form the arc. Arcs are measured in degrees. There are 360° around a circle.

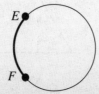

This is $\overset{\frown}{EF}$.

Minor $\overset{\frown}{EF}$ is shorter distance between *E* and *F*

Major $\overset{\frown}{EF}$ is longer distance between *E* and *F*

When $\overset{\frown}{EF}$ is written, the minor arc is assumed.

Circumference and Area

- *Circumference* is the distance around a circle. Since there are no sides to add up, a formula is needed. π (pi) is a Greek letter that represents a specific number. In fractional or decimal form, the commonly used approximations are: $\pi \approx 3.14$ or $\pi \approx \frac{22}{7}$.

   The formula for circumference is: $C = \pi d$ or $C = 2\pi r$.

   For example:

   In circle M, $d = 8$ because $r = 4$.

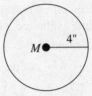

$$C = \pi d$$
$$= \pi(8)$$
$$= 3.14(8)$$
$$= 25.12 \text{ inches}$$

- The *area* of a circle can be determined by: $A = \pi r^2$.

   For example:

   In circle M, $r = 5$ because $d = 10$.

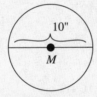

$$A = \pi(r^2)$$
$$= \pi(5^2)$$
$$= 3.14(25)$$
$$= 78.5 \text{ sq in}$$

Congruence and Similarity

Two plane (flat) geometric figures are said to be congruent if they are identical in size and shape. They are said to be similar if they have the same shape, but are not identical in size. For example:

All squares are similar.

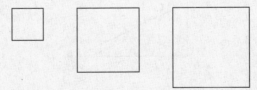

The following triangles are congruent.

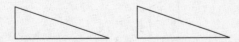

A more precise working definition of similar figures follows:

- Similar figures have corresponding angles equal and corresponding sides that are in proportion. Corresponding sides are those sides that are across from the equal angles.

For example:

Triangles *ADE* and *ACB* are similar

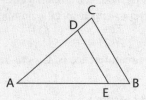

Side *DE* = 4 and corresponding

side *CB* = 6. If side *AD* = 6, then

side *AC* =

Since the triangles are similar, the corresponding sides are in proportion. The corresponding sides in the case are *AD* and *AC*, *DE* and *CB*, and *AE* and *AB*. The corresponding angles are ∠*DAE* and ∠*CAB*, ∠*ADE* and ∠*ACB*, and ∠*AED* and ∠*ABC*. Because the proportion of side *DE* to side CB is 4 to 6 or $\frac{4}{6}$, which reduces to $\frac{2}{3}$, the same ratio holds for all corresponding sides. Therefore,

$$\frac{AD}{AC} = \frac{DE}{CB} \text{ or } \frac{AD}{AC} = \frac{2}{3}$$

and since *AD* = 6, $\frac{6}{AC} = \frac{2}{3}$

Cross multiplying gives

$$6(3) = 2(AC)$$
$$18 = 2(AC)$$

Divide each side by 2.

$$\frac{18}{2} = \frac{2(AC)}{2}$$
$$9 = AC \text{ or } AC = 9$$

Please note that this question could have been introduced as follows:

In the triangle shown, *DE*∥*CB*. If *AD* = 4, *CB* = 6, and *AD* = 6, what is the length of *AC*?

A line parallel to one side within a triangle produces similar triangles. Therefore, triangles *ADE* and *ACB* are similar and the problem can be solved as above.

A few more examples:

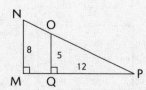

1. In the figure above, what is the length of PM?

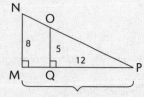

In the figure above, since MN and OQ are both perpendicular to PM, they are parallel to each other. Therefore, triangles OPQ and NPM are similar. Since OQ to NM is in the ratio 5 to 8, you can set up the following proportion to find PM.

$$\frac{OQ}{NM} = \frac{PQ}{PM} \text{ or } \frac{5}{8} = \frac{12}{PM}$$

Cross multiplying gives

$$5(PM) = 8(12)$$
$$5(PM) = 96$$

Divide each side by 5.

$$\frac{5(PM)}{5} = \frac{96}{5}$$
$$PM = 19\frac{1}{5} \text{ or } 19.2$$

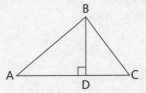

2. In the figure above, triangles $\angle ADB$ and $\angle BDC$ are similar. $\angle DAB = \angle DBC$, and $\angle ABD = \angle BCD$. What is the length of DC?

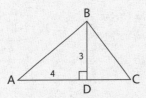

In the figure above, since triangles ADB and BDC are similar, the only real difficulty is matching the corresponding parts. Since $\angle BAD = \angle CBD$, they are corresponding and sides across from them, BD and DC, are corresponding. Since $\angle DCB = \angle DBA$, AD and BD are corresponding. (Note that BD is used twice, as it is part of both triangles.) Because BD to AD is in the ratio 3 to 4, you can set up the following proportion and solve accordingly.

$$\frac{BD}{AD} = \frac{DC}{BD} \text{ or } \frac{3}{4} = \frac{DC}{3}$$
$$3(3) = 4(DC)$$
$$9 = 4(DC)$$
$$\frac{9}{4} = \frac{4(DC)}{4}$$
$$2\frac{1}{4} = DC \text{ or } DC = 2\frac{1}{4} \text{ or } 2.25$$

Three-Dimensional Shapes

In three dimensions, additional facts can be determined about shapes.

Volume

Volume refers to the capacity to hold. The formula for volume of each shape is different.

The volume of any prism (a three-dimensional shape having many sides, but two bases) can be determined by:
Volume (V) = (area of base)(height of prism).

Specifically, for a rectangular solid:

$$V = (lw)(h)$$
$$= lwh$$

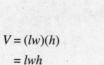

The formula for the volume of the cube
is often written $V = s \times s \times s = s^3$

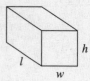

Specifically, for a cylinder (circular bases):

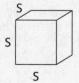

$$V = (\pi r^2)h$$
$$= \pi r^2 h$$

Volume is labeled in *cubic* units.

Some examples:

Find the volumes of the solid figures below with the dimensions indicated.

1. Rectangular Solid
   $V = lwh = (10)(5)(4) = 200$ cubic inches

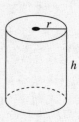

2. Cube
   $V = s^3 = 8 \times 8 \times 8 = 512$ cubic yards

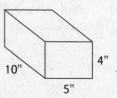

3. Cylinder
   $V = \pi r^2 h = \dfrac{22}{7} \times \dfrac{2}{1} \times \dfrac{2}{1} \times \dfrac{\cancel{14}^{2}}{1}$ $22(8) = 176$ cubic inches

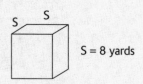

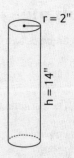

Surface Area

The surface area of a three-dimensional solid is the area of all the surfaces that form the solid. Find the area of each surface, and then add those areas. The surface area of a rectangular solid can be found by adding the areas of all six surfaces. For example:

The surface area of this prism is:

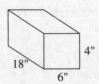

top:	$18 \times 6 = 108$
bottom:	$18 \times 6 = 108$
left side:	$6 \times 4 = 24$
right side:	$6 \times 4 = 24$
front:	$18 \times 4 = 72$
back:	$18 \times 4 = \underline{72}$
	408 sq in

To determine the *surface area of a right circular cylinder*, it is best envisioned "rolled out" onto a fat surface as below.

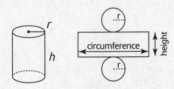

Now find the area of each individual piece. The area of each circle equals πr^2. Note that the length of the rectangle equals the circumference of the circle. The rectangle's area equals circumference times height. Adding the three parts gives the surface area of the cylinder. For example:

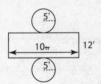

Find the surface area of a cylinder with radius 5' and height 12'.

The area of the circle $= \pi(r^2) = \pi(5^2) = 25\pi$.

The area of the bottom circle is the same, 25π.

The length of the rectangle is the circumference of the circle, or $2\pi r = 2\pi(5) = 10\pi$.

Therefore the area of the rectangle equals its height times $10\pi = 12 \times 10\pi = 120\pi$.

Totaling all the pieces gives $25\pi + 25\pi + 120\pi = 170\pi$.

Coordinate Geometry and Measurement

Refer to "Basic Coordinate Geometry" in the "Algebra Review" section if you need to review coordinate graphs.

Coordinate graphs can be used in measurement problems. For example:

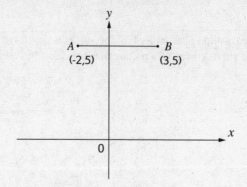

1. What is the length of *AB* in the preceding graph?

Since the coordinates of the points are (–2, 5) and (3, 5), the first, or *x*-coordinate is the clue to the distance of each point from the *y*-axis. The distance to point B from the *y*-axis is 3, and the distance to point A from the *y*-axis is 2. (–2 is 2 in the negative direction.) So 3 + 2 gives a length of 5.

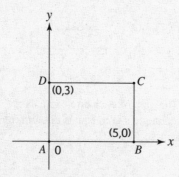

2. What is the area of rectangle *ABCD* in the preceding graph?

The formula for the area of a rectangle is base × height. Since point A is at (0, 0) and point B is at (5, 0), the base is 5. Since point D is at (0, 3), the height is 3, so the area is 5 × 3 = 15.

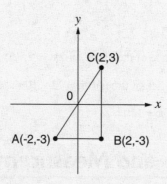

3. What is the area of △*ABC* in the preceding figure?

The area of a triangle is $\frac{1}{2}$ × base × height.

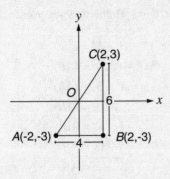

Base *AB* of the triangle is 4 units (because from *A* to the *y*-axis is 2 units and from the *y*-axis to *B* is another 2 units). Height *BC* of the triangle is 6 units (3 units from *B* to the *x*-axis and another 3 units to *C*). Note that $\angle B$ is a right angle. So

$$\text{area of triangle} = \frac{1}{2} \times 4 \times 6$$
$$= \frac{1}{2} \times 24$$
$$= 12$$

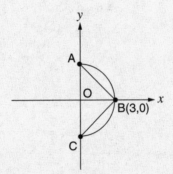

4. In the preceding figure, what is the perimeter of $\triangle ABC$ inscribed within the semicircle with center *O*?

To find the perimeter of the triangle, you need the lengths of the three sides. You know that radius *OB* is 3 units long. The *OA* and *OC* are each 3 units because they are also radii. Therefore, side *AC* of the triangle is 6 units.

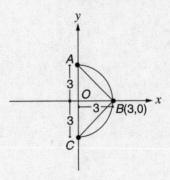

In triangle AOB, you know that OA is 3 and OB is 3. From the Pythagorean theorem,

$$a^2 + b^2 = c^2$$
$$(OA)^2 + (OB)^2 = (AB)^2$$
$$3^2 + 3^2 = (AB)^2$$
$$9 + 9 = (AB)^2$$
$$18 = AB^2$$
$$\sqrt{18} = AB$$
$$\sqrt{9 \times 2} = AB$$
$$3\sqrt{2} = AB$$

(If you spotted that triangle AOB is an isosceles right triangle with sides in the ratio $1 : 1 : \sqrt{2}$, you wouldn't have needed to use the Pythagorean theorem.)

By symmetry, you know that $AB = CB$. So $CB = 3\sqrt{2}$ and

$$\text{perimeter} = CA + AB + CB$$
$$= 6 + 3\sqrt{2} + 3\sqrt{2}$$
$$= 6 + 6\sqrt{2}$$

PART III

TWO SIMULATED ELM PRACTICE TESTS

The ELM has 50 multiple-choice questions, but only 45 actually count toward your score. The 5 additional questions, which can be scattered throughout the exam, are being tested for future exams. Each practice test in this section has 50 questions, followed by complete explanations.

Remember, the time limit on the ELM is 90 minutes.

The problems in these simulated practice exams are designed to be similar in structure, style, variety, and difficulty level to the problems on the actual exam. There may be some variance from exam to exam. The actual ELM is copyrighted and may not be duplicated. These questions are not taken from the actual tests.

Answer Sheet for Practice Test 1

(Remove This Sheet and Use It to Mark Your Answers)

1 Ⓐ Ⓑ Ⓒ Ⓓ	26 Ⓐ Ⓑ Ⓒ Ⓓ
2 Ⓐ Ⓑ Ⓒ Ⓓ	27 Ⓐ Ⓑ Ⓒ Ⓓ
3 Ⓐ Ⓑ Ⓒ Ⓓ	28 Ⓐ Ⓑ Ⓒ Ⓓ
4 Ⓐ Ⓑ Ⓒ Ⓓ	29 Ⓐ Ⓑ Ⓒ Ⓓ
5 Ⓐ Ⓑ Ⓒ Ⓓ	30 Ⓐ Ⓑ Ⓒ Ⓓ
6 Ⓐ Ⓑ Ⓒ Ⓓ	31 Ⓐ Ⓑ Ⓒ Ⓓ
7 Ⓐ Ⓑ Ⓒ Ⓓ	32 Ⓐ Ⓑ Ⓒ Ⓓ
8 Ⓐ Ⓑ Ⓒ Ⓓ	33 Ⓐ Ⓑ Ⓒ Ⓓ
9 Ⓐ Ⓑ Ⓒ Ⓓ	34 Ⓐ Ⓑ Ⓒ Ⓓ
10 Ⓐ Ⓑ Ⓒ Ⓓ	35 Ⓐ Ⓑ Ⓒ Ⓓ
11 Ⓐ Ⓑ Ⓒ Ⓓ	36 Ⓐ Ⓑ Ⓒ Ⓓ
12 Ⓐ Ⓑ Ⓒ Ⓓ	37 Ⓐ Ⓑ Ⓒ Ⓓ
13 Ⓐ Ⓑ Ⓒ Ⓓ	38 Ⓐ Ⓑ Ⓒ Ⓓ
14 Ⓐ Ⓑ Ⓒ Ⓓ	39 Ⓐ Ⓑ Ⓒ Ⓓ
15 Ⓐ Ⓑ Ⓒ Ⓓ	40 Ⓐ Ⓑ Ⓒ Ⓓ
16 Ⓐ Ⓑ Ⓒ Ⓓ	41 Ⓐ Ⓑ Ⓒ Ⓓ
17 Ⓐ Ⓑ Ⓒ Ⓓ	42 Ⓐ Ⓑ Ⓒ Ⓓ
18 Ⓐ Ⓑ Ⓒ Ⓓ	43 Ⓐ Ⓑ Ⓒ Ⓓ
19 Ⓐ Ⓑ Ⓒ Ⓓ	44 Ⓐ Ⓑ Ⓒ Ⓓ
20 Ⓐ Ⓑ Ⓒ Ⓓ	45 Ⓐ Ⓑ Ⓒ Ⓓ
21 Ⓐ Ⓑ Ⓒ Ⓓ	46 Ⓐ Ⓑ Ⓒ Ⓓ
22 Ⓐ Ⓑ Ⓒ Ⓓ	47 Ⓐ Ⓑ Ⓒ Ⓓ
23 Ⓐ Ⓑ Ⓒ Ⓓ	48 Ⓐ Ⓑ Ⓒ Ⓓ
24 Ⓐ Ⓑ Ⓒ Ⓓ	49 Ⓐ Ⓑ Ⓒ Ⓓ
25 Ⓐ Ⓑ Ⓒ Ⓓ	50 Ⓐ Ⓑ Ⓒ Ⓓ

CUT HERE

CUT HERE

Geometry Reference Formulas

CUT HERE

Rectangle

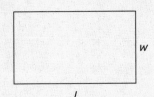

Area = lw
Perimeter = $2l + 2w$

Triangle

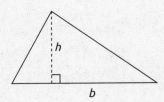

Area = $\frac{1}{2}bh$

Circle

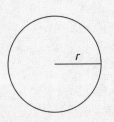

Area = πr^2
Circumference = $2\pi r$

Rectangular Solid

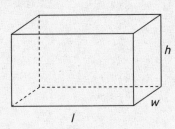

Volume = lwh

Right Circular Cylinder

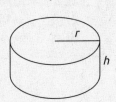

Volume = $\pi r^2 h$

Pythagorean Theorem

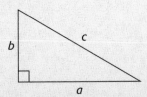

$c^2 = a^2 + b^2$

CUT HERE

90 Minutes

50 Questions

Directions: Solve for each of the following problems. You may use the blank space for scratchwork.

Notes: (1) Unless otherwise specified, the denominators of algebraic expressions appearing in these problems are assumed to be nonzero. (2) Figures that accompany problems are drawn as accurately as possible EXCEPT when it is stated that a figure is not drawn to scale. (3) The Geometry Reference Formulas appearing on the previous page will be printed inside the front cover of the ELM test book.

---

1. If $x = -2$, then $2x^2 - x =$

   A.   6
   B.   10
   C.   16
   D.   18
   E.   20

3. The square root of 200 is between

   A.   12 and 13
   B.   13 and 14
   C.   14 and 15
   D.   15 and 16
   E.   16 and 17

Airspeed

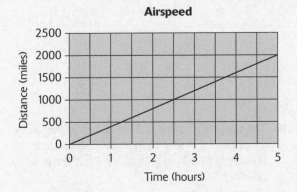

Distance (miles) vs Time (hours)

2. According to the graph above, how fast is the airplane flying in miles per hour?

   A.   300
   B.   400
   C.   500
   D.   600
   E.   700

4. Ramon is paid $7 per hour (after taxes are deducted) and puts 20% of his earnings in a savings account. How many hours will he have to work in order to have enough money in his savings account to purchase a coat that sells for $77?

   A.   9
   B.   11
   C.   55
   D.   305
   E.   360

GO ON TO THE NEXT PAGE

5. $\sqrt{9x^{16}} =$

   A.   3

   B. $3x^4$

   C. $3x^8$

   D. $3x^{16}$

   E. $3x^{18}$

6. What is the area of a circle whose circumference is 20π?

   A. 10π

   B. 20π

   C. 40π

   D. 50π

   E. 100π

**Celia's Homework Schedule:
3 hours total**

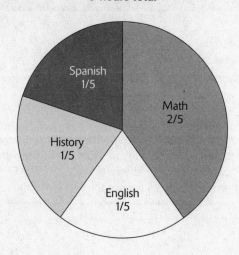

7. According to her schedule, how much time should Celia spend on her math homework?

   A.   24 minutes

   B.   36 minutes

   C.   72 minutes

   D.   96 minutes

   E.   108 minutes

8. The price of gasoline in June is 20% higher than the price of gasoline in January. If the price in January is $1.50 per gallon, what will the price in June be?

   A. $1.20

   B. $1.70

   C. $1.75

   D. $1.80

   E. $2.10

9. Which equation is the same as $\frac{x}{5} - \frac{2}{3} = 6$?

    A. $3x - 10 = 90$
    B. $5x - 6 = 90$
    C. $3x - 6 = 6$
    D. $5x - 6 = 6$
    E. $5x + 6 = 6$

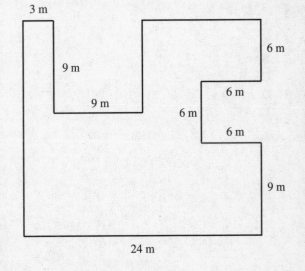

10. $2y - 1 < -5$ is equivalent to

    A. $y < -2$
    B. $y > -2$
    C. $y < 2$
    D. $y > 2$
    E. $y > 3$

11. All the angles shown in the figure above are right angles. What is the area of the figure?

    A. 387 square meters
    B. 468 square meters
    C. 504 square meters
    D. 576 square meters
    E. 567 square meters

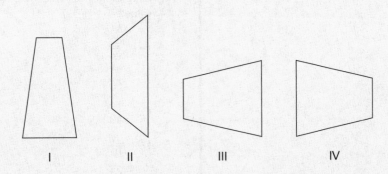

12. Which two of the figures above are congruent?

    A. I and II
    B. I and III
    C. II and III
    D. II and IV
    E. III and IV

GO ON TO THE NEXT PAGE

13. $\dfrac{3^3}{3^{-2}} =$

    A. 3^{-6}

    B. $3^{-1.5}$

    C. 3

    D. 3^5

    E. 3^6

14. If $\dfrac{3}{3x+3} = \dfrac{2}{x-1}$, then $x =$

    A. 9

    B. 6

    C. 3

    D. 0

    E. −3

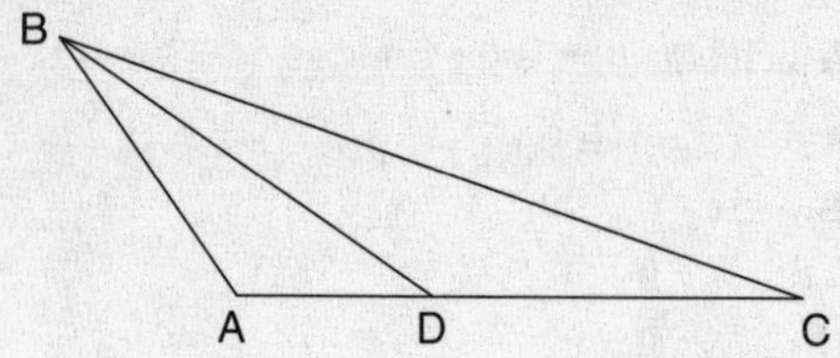

15. In the figure, $AB = AD$ and $BD = CD$. If $\angle C$ measures 19°, what is the measure of $\angle A$ in degrees?

    A. 75

    B. 94

    C. 104

    D. 142

    E. 184

16. Of the following fractions, which is the largest in value?

    A. $\dfrac{25}{52}$

    B. $\dfrac{31}{60}$

    C. $\dfrac{19}{40}$

    D. $\dfrac{51}{103}$

    E. $\dfrac{43}{90}$

17. If $f(x) = 2x^2 - 5x - 1$, then $f(-1) =$

    A.   −7

    B.   −6

    C.   3

    D.   4

    E.   6

18. A girl runs k miles in n hours. How many miles will she run in x hours at the same rate?

    A. knx

    B. $\dfrac{k}{n}$

    C. $\dfrac{kx}{n}$

    D. kx

    E. $\dfrac{kn}{x}$

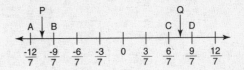

19. In the number line shown above, point P is midway between A and B. Point Q is midway between C and D. What is the distance between points P and Q?

    A. $\dfrac{3}{7}$

    B. $\dfrac{4}{7}$

    C. $\dfrac{6}{7}$

    D. $\dfrac{17}{7}$

    E. $\dfrac{18}{7}$

20. Which of the following is equivalent to $\dfrac{\left(2ab^2\right)\left(3a^2b\right)}{ab}$?

    A. $5ab$

    B. $6ab$

    C. $5a^2b^2$

    D. $6a^2b$

    E. $6a^2b^2$

GO ON TO THE NEXT PAGE

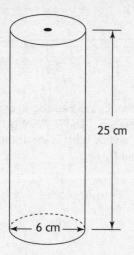

25 cm

6 cm

21. A national brand of potato chips is sold in a cylindrical container with dimensions as shown above.

What is the approximate volume of this potato chip container?

A. 236 cm³
B. 707 cm³
C. 942 cm³
D. 2,826 cm³
E. 3,680 cm³

Month	Rainfall (in inches)
January	3.6
February	3.6
March	2.7
April	3.1
May	2.0

22. The rainfall for 5 months is shown in the table above. What was the mean rainfall for the period?

A. 3.0 inches
B. 3.1 inches
C. 3.6 inches
D. 15.0 inches
E. 16.0 inches

23. Which of the following points lies on the line $2y = 3x - 4$?

A. $(0, -2)$
B. $(2, 3)$
C. $(3, 2)$
D. $(3, 5)$
E. $(2, 5)$

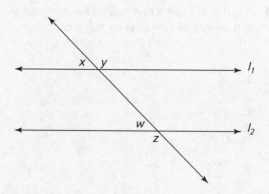

24. In the figure above, l_1 is parallel to l_2 and $x = 45°$. What is the value of w?

A. 45°
B. 90°
C. 135°
D. 180°
E. 225°

126

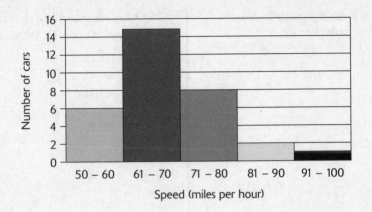

Speed (miles per hour)

25. The preceding graph shows the number of cars on a freeway traveling at the indicated speeds. How many cars are traveling faster than 70 miles per hour?

    A.   8 cars

    B.   10 cars

    C.   11 cars

    D.   26 cars

    E.   27 cars

26. What is the solution set for the equation $|3x - 3| = 15$?

    A. $\{-4\}$

    B. $\{6\}$

    C. $\{-4, 6\}$

    D. $\{-6, 6\}$

    E. $\{4, -6\}$

28. A bullet train has completed 300 miles of a 750-mile trip in 40 minutes. If it continues to travel at the same speed, how long will it take to complete the trip?

    A.   60 minutes

    B.   80 minutes

    C.   100 minutes

    D.   120 minutes

    E.   140 minutes

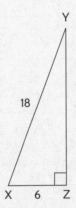 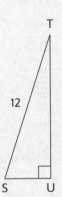

27. Triangles *XYZ* and *STU* in the figure above are similar. What is the length of *SU*?

    A.   10

    B.   9

    C.   8

    D.   4

    E.   3

GO ON TO THE NEXT PAGE

29. If the edge of a cube is multiplied by 3, then the volume of the cube is multiplied by

    A.   3
    B.   6
    C.   9
    D.   18
    E.   27

31. Janet has taken four tests in French class, scoring 62, 85, 90, and 75. What is her median score?

    A.   78
    B.   80
    C.   87.5
    D.   90
    E.   92.5

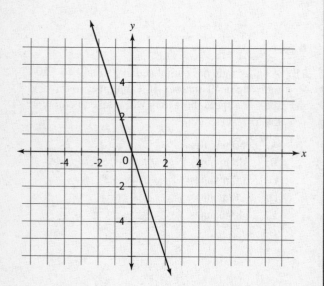

30. What is the slope of the line shown in the graph above?

    A.   −3
    B. $-\frac{1}{3}$
    C. $\frac{1}{3}$
    D.   3
    E.   4

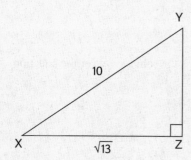

32. In the right triangle *XYZ* above, *YZ* =

    A. $\sqrt{170}$
    B.   13
    C. $\sqrt{113}$
    D.   10
    E. $\sqrt{87}$

33. $\dfrac{6}{5t} - \dfrac{2}{t} =$

   A. $\dfrac{4}{t}$

   B. $\dfrac{16}{5t}$

   C. $-\dfrac{2}{t}$

   D. $-\dfrac{2}{5t}$

   E. $-\dfrac{4}{5t}$

35. The value 68% falls between which one of the following pairs of fractions?

   A. $\dfrac{3}{8}$ and $\dfrac{2}{5}$

   B. $\dfrac{3}{5}$ and $\dfrac{5}{6}$

   C. $\dfrac{1}{2}$ and $\dfrac{2}{3}$

   D. $\dfrac{7}{10}$ and $\dfrac{3}{4}$

   E. $\dfrac{4}{5}$ and $\dfrac{9}{10}$

34. Line A is parallel to a line that has a slope of $\dfrac{1}{2}$. Which of the following could be the equation for line A?

   A. $y = -2x + 4$

   B. $y = \dfrac{1}{2}x + 4$

   C. $y = x + \dfrac{1}{2}$

   D. $y = 2x + 4$

   E. $y = x + 3$

36. Alice wants to send 400 wedding invitations. She can do about 16 per day. If she begins on January 1, when would she be expected to be finished?

   A. January 25

   B. February 18

   C. March 30

   D. April 15

   E. May 1

GO ON TO THE NEXT PAGE

37. What is the solution to $x - 1 \geq |2 - 4|$?

    A. $x > -1$

    B. $x \geq -1$

    C. $x > 3$

    D. $x \geq 3$

    E. $x \geq 2$

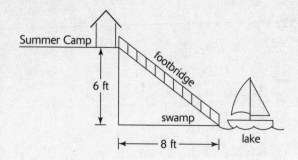

39. As shown in the diagram above, camp counselor Craig build a footbridge from the summer camp to the lake so that the campers would not have to crawl down a perpendicular 6-foot cliff and then trudge through 8 feet of swamp.

How long is the footbridge?

    A.   14 feet

    B.   12 feet

    C.   11 feet

    D.   10 feet

    E.   9 feet

38. What is the solution to the following system of equations?

$$\begin{cases} 6x - 2y = 4 \\ 2x + y = 8 \end{cases}$$

    A. $(-4, 2)$

    B. $(-2, 4)$

    C. $(2, 4)$

    D. $(4, 2)$

    E. $(-2, -4)$

40. There are 36 students in a certain geometry class. If $\frac{2}{3}$ of the students are boys and $\frac{3}{4}$ of the boys are under 6 feet tall, how many boys in the class are under 6 feet tall?

    A.   6

    B.   12

    C.   18

    D.   24

    E.   27

41. The base of an isosceles triangle exceeds each of the equal sides by 8 feet. If the perimeter is 89 feet, what is the length of the base?

   A.   27 feet

   B. $29\frac{2}{3}$ feet

   C.   35 feet

   D.   54 feet

   E.   70 feet

42. Joe needs to buy 90 tiles; each tile costs $2.15. He estimates the total cost to be about $2,000. Which of the following statements is correct?

   A.   Joe's estimate is about one-tenth of the exact cost.

   B.   Joe's estimate is very close to the exact cost.

   C.   Joe's estimate is about 10 times the exact cost.

   D.   Joe's estimate is about 100 times the exact cost.

   E.   Joe's estimate is about 1,000 times the exact cost.

43. If $\frac{5}{4} = 3y + \frac{1}{4}$, then $y =$

   A. $\frac{1}{3}$

   B. $\frac{1}{2}$

   C. $\frac{3}{4}$

   D.   3

   E.   4

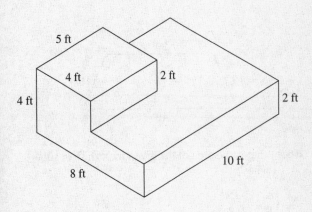

44. What is the volume of the shape above?

   A.   200 ft^3

   B.   240 ft^3

   C.   360 ft^3

   D.   400 ft^3

   E.   420 ft^3

GO ON TO THE NEXT PAGE

45. Tom counts the change in his pocket: He has $\frac{1}{2}$ of a dollar, $\frac{3}{4}$ of a dollar, $\frac{3}{10}$ of a dollar, $\frac{3}{20}$ of a a dollar, and $\frac{1}{50}$ of a dollar. How much change does Tom have?

   A. $1.42
   B. $1.72
   C. $2.00
   D. $2.60
   E. $2.72

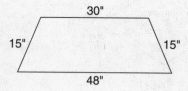

46. What is the area of the given trapezoid, in square inches?

   A. 585
   B. 468
   C. 234
   D. 108
   E.   78

47. The Tigers have won 75% of their baseball games. How many of the 32 remaining games can they lose and still maintain their current winning percentage?

   A. 8
   B. 16
   C. 24
   D. 25
   E. 26

48. Which of the following expressions represents the statement, "four less than one-third the product of 10 and n"?

   A. $\frac{10+n}{3} - 4$

   B. $\frac{10n}{3} - 4$

   C. $\frac{1}{3}(10n - 4)$

   D. $\frac{1}{3}(10 + n - 4)$

   E. $4 - \frac{1}{3}10n$

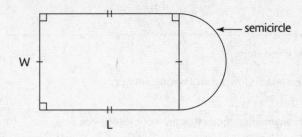

← semicircle

W

L

49. Which equation represents the total area, A, of the figure above?

A. $LW + \left(\dfrac{\pi}{2}\right)W^2$

B. $W + 2L + 2\pi W$

C. $LW + \left(\dfrac{\pi}{8}\right)W^2$

D. $LW + \pi W$

E. $LW + 2\pi$

50. The point $(3, 7)$ lies on a line that has a slope of 1. What is the y-intercept of the line?

A. $(0, -4)$

B. $(-4, 0)$

C. $(0, 4)$

D. $(4, 0)$

E. $(4, -4)$

IF YOU FINISH BEFORE TIME IS CALLED, CHECK YOUR WORK ON THIS SECTION ONLY. DO NOT WORK ON ANY OTHER SECTION IN THE TEST.

Reviewing Practice Test 1

Review your simulated ELM Practice Examination by following these steps:

1. Check the Answer Key that follows. Put a checkmark in the box following any wrong answer.
2. Fill out the Review Chart (page 136).
3. Read all explanations (pages 137–145). Go back to review any explanations that are not clear to you.
4. Fill out the Reasons for Mistakes chart on page 136.
5. Go back to the math review section and review any basic skills necessary before taking the next practice test.

Don't leave out any of these steps. They are very important in learning to do your best on the ELM.

Answer Key for Practice Test 1

(Number Sense – NS) (Algebra – Al) (Geometry – G)

1. B ❑ (Al)
2. B ❑ (NS)
3. C ❑ (NS)
4. C ❑ (NS)
5. C ❑ (Al)
6. E ❑ (G)
7. C ❑ (NS)
8. D ❑ (NS)
9. A ❑ (Al)
10. A ❑ (Al)
11. A ❑ (G)
12. E ❑ (G)
13. D ❑ (Al)
14. E ❑ (Al)
15. C ❑ (G)
16. B ❑ (NS)
17. E ❑ (Al)
18. C ❑ (NS)
19. E ❑ (NS)
20. E ❑ (Al)
21. B ❑ (G)
22. A ❑ (NS)
23. A ❑ (Al)
24. A ❑ (G)
25. C ❑ (NS)

26. C ❑ (Al)
27. D ❑ (G)
28. A ❑ (NS)
29. E ❑ (G)
30. A ❑ (Al)
31. B ❑ (NS)
32. E ❑ (G)
33. E ❑ (Al)
34. B ❑ (Al)
35. B ❑ (NS)
36. A ❑ (NS)
37. D ❑ (Al)
38. C ❑ (Al)
39. D ❑ (G)
40. C ❑ (NS)
41. C ❑ (G)
42. C ❑ (NS)
43. A ❑ (Al)
44. A ❑ (G)
45. B ❑ (NS)
46. B ❑ (G)
47. A ❑ (NS)
48. B ❑ (Al)
49. C ❑ (G)
50. C ❑ (Al)

Review Chart

Use your marked Answer Key to fill in the following chart for the multiple-choice questions.

	Possible	Completed	Right	Wrong
Number Sense (NS)	18			
Algebra (Al)	18			
Geometry (G)	14			
Totals	50			

Reasons for Mistakes

Fill out the following chart only after you have read all the explanations that follow. This chart will help you spot your strengths and weaknesses and your repeated errors or trends in types of errors.

	Total Missed	Simple Mistake	Misread Problem	Lack of Knowledge
Number Sense (NS)				
Algebra (Al)				
Geometry (G)				
Totals				

Examine your results carefully. Reviewing the above information will help you pinpoint your common mistakes. Focus on avoiding your most common mistakes as you practice. The "Lack of Knowledge" column will help you focus your review in the math review section. If you are missing a lot of questions because of "Lack of Knowledge," you should go back and spend extra time reviewing the basics.

Answer Explanations for Practice Test 1

1. B. To solve this problem, rewrite the expression by substituting –2 in place of x.

$$2x^2 - x$$
$$2(-2)^2 - (-2)$$

Then perform the operations in the appropriate order.

To do that, remember:

Parentheses
Exponents
Multiplication $\Big\}$ Left to right, whichever comes first
Division
Addition $\Big\}$ Left to right, whichever comes first
Subtraction

So, you must first square –2:

$$2(4) - (-2)$$

Next you must multiply:

$$8 - (-2)$$

Finally, subtract –2:

$$8 - (-2) = 10$$

2. B. The easiest way to solve this problem is to look for a place where the graphed line crosses an intersection on the grid. This happens at 2.5 hours, and at 5 hours. At the 5-hour mark, the airplane has traveled 2,000 miles.

$$2,000 \div 5 = 400$$

3. C. The square root of 144 is 12 because $12 \times 12 = 144$. Likewise,

The square root of 169 is 13.

The square root of 196 is 14.

The square root of 225 is 15.

The square root of 256 is 16.

Two hundred is between 196 and 225; therefore, the square root of 200 is between 14 and 15.

4. C. For each hour he works, Ramon saves 20% of $7.00, or $1.40 per hour. So to purchase a $77 coat from his savings, he will need to work $\frac{\$77}{\$1.40/\text{hr}} = 55$ hours; thus Choice C is correct.

5. C. The square root of 9 is 3 because $3 \times 3 = 9$. The square root of x^{16} is x^8 because $(x^8)(x^8) = x^{16}$. Therefore, $\sqrt{9x^{16}} = 3x^8$.

6. E. Since the formula for area of a circle is $A = \pi r^2$, and the circumference formula is $C = 2\pi r$, first use the circumference formula to solve for the radius.

$$C = 20\pi$$
$$2\pi r = 20\pi$$
$$\frac{2\pi r}{2\pi} = \frac{20\pi}{2\pi}$$
$$r = 10$$

137

Now plug the radius of 10 into the area formula.

$$A = \pi r^2$$
$$A = \pi (10)^2$$
$$A = 100\pi$$

7. C. Celia spends $\frac{2}{5}$ of her homework time on math, so you must find $\frac{2}{5}$ of 3 hours. Since the answer choices are expressed in minutes, convert 3 hours to 180 minutes, and find $\frac{2}{5}$ of 180 minutes:

$$\frac{2}{5} \times 180 = 72 \text{ minutes}$$

8. D. Twenty percent of $1.50 = .2 \times \$1.50 = \$.30$. So, the price increases $.30 from January to June. Thirty cents more than $1.50 is $1.80.

9. A. To clear the fractions on the left side of the equation, multiply each side of the equation by the least common denominator of the fractions. The least common denominator of 5 and 3 is 15, so:

$$\frac{x}{5} - \frac{2}{3} = 6$$
$$15\left(\frac{x}{5} - \frac{2}{3}\right) = 15(6)$$
$$\frac{15 \cdot x}{5} - \frac{15 \cdot 2}{3} = 90$$
$$3x - 10 = 90$$

10. A. To solve this inequality:

$$2y - 1 < -5$$
$$\underline{+1 = +1} \qquad \text{Add 1 to each side to isolate the variable.}$$
$$2y \quad < -4$$
$$\frac{2y}{2} \quad < \frac{-4}{2} \qquad \text{Divide each side by 2 to clear the coefficient.}$$
$$y \quad < -2$$

11. A. A simple way to solve this is to find the area of a larger rectangle and subtract the two pieces that are not part of the irregular figure. The dimensions of the larger rectangle are 24 meters by 21 meters; its area is 24 meters $\times$ 21 meters = 504 square meters. From this, subtract the two smaller areas: 9 meters $\times$ 9 meters = 81 square meters, and 6 meters $\times$ 6 meters = 36 square meters. $504 - (81 + 36) = 387$ meters.

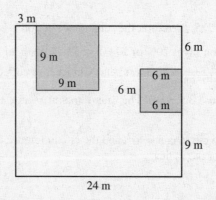

12. E. Congruent means exactly the same. Notice that III and IV are mirror images of each other.

13. D. To divide common bases with exponents, you subtract the exponents:

$$\frac{3^3}{3^{-2}} = 3^{3-(-2)} = 3^5$$

14. E. Simply cross multiply; $\frac{3}{3x+3} = \frac{2}{x-1}$ gives $3x - 3 = 6x + 6$. Next solve for x as follows:

Subtract $3x$,
$$3x - 3 = 6x + 6$$
$$\underline{-3x \qquad -3x}$$
$$-3 = 3x + 6$$

Subtract 6,
$$\underline{-6 \qquad -6}$$
$$-9 = 3x$$

Now divide by 3,
$$\frac{-9}{3} = \frac{3x}{3}$$
$$-3 = x$$

15. C. Since $BD = CD$, $\angle CBD = \angle C = 19°$

$$\text{Hence } \angle BCD = 180 - (\angle CBD + \angle C)$$
$$= 180 - (19 + 19)$$
$$= 180 - 38$$
$$\angle BDC = 142°$$

$$\text{Then } \angle BDA = 180 - \angle BDC$$
$$= 180 - 142$$
$$\angle BDA = 38°$$

Since $AB = AD$, $\angle ABD = \angle BDA = 38°$

$$\text{Hence } \angle A = 180 - (\angle BDA + \angle ABD)$$
$$= 180 - (38 + 38)$$
$$= 180 - 76$$
$$\angle A = 104°$$

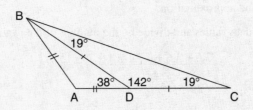

16. B. Only Choice B, $\frac{31}{60}$, is greater than $\frac{1}{2}$. All the other choices are less than $\frac{1}{2}$.

17. E. In place of x, simply plug in -1 into $2x^2 - 5x - 1$.

$$2(-1)^2 - 5(-1) - 1$$
$$2(1) + 5 - 1$$
$$2 + 5 - 1 = 6$$

18. C. Distance = rate × time:

$$d = rt$$
$$k = rn$$
$$r = \frac{k}{n} \text{ miles per hour}$$
$$d = \frac{k}{n}(x) = \frac{kx}{n}$$

19. E. Each tick mark is $\frac{3}{7}$ unit wide. Point P is 3.5 tick marks away from 0, and point Q is 2.5 tick marks away from 0. Therefore, the total distance between P and Q is 2.5 + 3.5 = 6 tick marks. Since each tick mark is $\frac{3}{7}$ unit, the total distance is $6 \times \frac{3}{7} = \frac{18}{7}$.

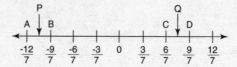

20. E. To simplify this fractional expression, multiply the terms in the numerator and divide by the term in the denominator:

$$\frac{\left(2ab^2\right)\left(3a^2b\right)}{ab}$$

$$\frac{(2 \cdot 3)(a \cdot a \cdot a)(b \cdot b \cdot b)}{ab} =$$

$$\frac{a}{a} \cdot \frac{b}{b} \cdot (2 \cdot 3)(a \cdot a)(b \cdot b) =$$

$$1 \times 1(6a^2b^2) = 6a^2b^2$$

Just realizing that you are going to multiply 2 by 3 to get 6 allows you to eliminate choices A and C.

21. B. The formula for the volume of a right circular cylinder is $V = \pi r^2 h$.

Since the diameter of the cylinder is 6 cm, its radius is 3 cm. Then the volume is: $V = (3.14)(3^2)(25) = 706.5$ cm^3

So 707 cm^3, Choice B, is a good approximation.

22. A. To find the mean, add the data values and divide by the number of data values:

$$\frac{3.6 + 3.6 + 2.7 + 3.1 + 2}{5} = \frac{15}{5} = 3$$

So, the mean is 3 inches.

23. A. If the point lies on the line, then it must satisfy the equation of the line. Substitute the answer choices into the given equation until you find the one that works. Fortunately, it might be the first one you try, Choice A:

$$2y = 3x - 4$$
$$2(-2) = (3)(0) - 4$$
$$-4 = -4$$

That is true, so the point (0, −2) lies on the line.

24. A. Since $x = 45°$, then $y = 135°$ (they form a straight line). All of the angles are either 45° or 135°. Since x corresponds to w, then $w = 45°$.

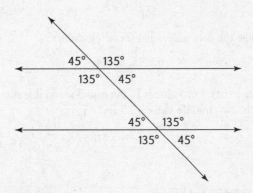

25. C. You're looking only for cars traveling faster than 70 miles per hour. These are represented in the graph by three bars. Eight cars are traveling between 71 and 80 miles per hour; two cars are traveling between 81 and 90 miles per hour; one car is traveling between 91 and 100 miles per hour. $8 + 2 + 1 = 11$

26. C. The easiest way to deal with an absolute value equation like this might be to substitute the answer choices into the equation and see which ones work. Absolute value is always positive, so the total quantity within the absolute value bars can be positive or negative.

What makes this equation tricky is that the entire left side of the equation is enclosed within absolute value bars. In essence, what it's saying is that $3x - 3$ is equal to either 15, or to –15. So you need to solve two equations:

$$3x - 3 = 15 \qquad\qquad 3x - 3 = -15$$
$$\underline{+3 = +3} \qquad\qquad\quad \underline{+3 = +3}$$
$$3x = 18 \qquad\qquad\quad 3x = -12$$
$$\frac{3x}{3} = \frac{18}{3} \qquad\qquad\quad \frac{3x}{3} = \frac{-12}{3}$$
$$x = 6 \qquad\qquad\qquad x = -4$$

27. D. Since the triangles are similar, the corresponding sides are in proportion. Simply set up the ratio as follows and solve.

$$\frac{6}{18} = \frac{SU}{12}$$

Reduce $\qquad\qquad \dfrac{1}{3} = \dfrac{SU}{12}$

Cross multiply $\qquad 12 = 3SU$

Divide by 3 $\qquad\quad 4 = SU$

28. A. Be careful on this kind of problem! It's not difficult, but you need to read it carefully. In this case, we're not looking for the time required for the entire trip—for the rest of it. The entire trip is 750 miles, and 300 miles have been completed—so 450 miles remain. Four hundred and fifty is one-and-a-half times as big as 300, so it takes one-and-a-half times as long as 40 minutes, which is an hour. Or you could set up the following proportion and solve for x:

$$\frac{40}{300} = \frac{x}{450}$$

29. E. Try a simple example. If the edge of a cube is 1, then the volume is $1 \times 1 \times 1 = 1$. If the edge of a cube is 3, then the volume is $3 \times 3 \times 3 = 27$. So the volume is multiplied by 27.

30. A. Since the line slopes downward from left to right, it has a negative slope; therefore, you can eliminate choices C, D, and E. Remember that slope is defined as:

$$\frac{\text{vertical shift}}{\text{horizontal shift}}$$

In this case, the line goes down three units for every unit it moves to the right:

$$\frac{-3}{1} = -3$$

31. B. To find the median, rearrange the data values in ascending order:

$$62, 75, 85, 90$$

If an odd number of data values exists, one value is in the middle, and it is the median. However, in this case, the median lies halfway between the two middle values, 75 and 85.

$$\frac{75 + 85}{2} = 80$$

So, 80 is the median.

32. E. Plug into the Pythagorean theorem as follows:

$$a^2 + b^2 = c^2$$
$$\left(\sqrt{13}\right)^2 + b^2 = (10)^2$$
$$13 + b^2 = 100$$
$$\underline{-13 \quad -13}$$
$$b^2 = 87$$
$$b = \sqrt{87}$$

33. E. Since the LCD is $5t$, simply multiply the second term by 5 and then subtract the numerators and keep the LCD.

$$\frac{6}{5t} - \frac{2(5)}{t(5)} =$$

$$\frac{6}{5t} - \frac{10}{5t} = -\frac{4}{5t}$$

34. B. Lines that are parallel have the same slope. All the answer choices are expressed in the slope-intercept form, $y = mx + b$, where m is the slope. Choice B is the only answer that has a slope of $\frac{1}{2}$.

35. B. The process of elimination will help you find the correct answer. Note that the bigger fraction in Choice A is only $\frac{2}{5}$, or 40%. Thus, Choice A is incorrect. In Choice C, $\frac{1}{2}$ is 50% and $\frac{2}{3}$ is $66\frac{2}{3}$%. Thus, Choice C is incorrect. In Choice D, $\frac{7}{10}$ is 70% and $\frac{3}{4}$ is 75%. Thus, Choice D is incorrect. And Choice E is between 80% and 90%. Choice B is correct: $\frac{3}{5}$ is 60%, and $\frac{5}{6}$ is $83\frac{1}{3}$%. Thus, 68% lies between them.

36. A. You want to find how many groups of 16 it takes to make 400, so divide 16 into 400.

$$\begin{array}{r} 25 \\ 16\overline{)400} \\ \underline{32} \\ 80 \\ \underline{80} \\ 0 \end{array}$$

So it would take 25 days.

37. D. To solve this inequality:

$$x - 1 \geq |2 - 4|$$
$$x - 1 \geq |-2|$$
$$x - 1 \geq 2$$
$$\underline{+1 = +1} \qquad \text{Add 1 to each side to isolate the variable.}$$
$$x \geq 3$$

38. C. If you are unfamiliar with techniques for solving a system of equations, the easiest way to solve this problem is to substitute the coordinates given as answer choices in the equations until you find a choice that works in both equations. That is Choice C:

$$6(2) - 2(4) = 4$$
$$2(2) + 4 = 8$$

39. D. To solve this, you need to find the hypotenuse (the footbridge) of the right triangle by using the Pythagorean theorem:

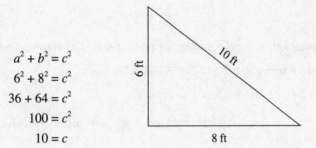

$$a^2 + b^2 = c^2$$
$$6^2 + 8^2 = c^2$$
$$36 + 64 = c^2$$
$$100 = c^2$$
$$10 = c$$

40. C. Since $\frac{2}{3}$ of the students are boys, there are $\frac{2}{3}(36) = 24$ boys in the class. Out of the 24 boys in the class, $\frac{3}{4}$ are under 6 feet tall, or $\frac{3}{4}(24) = 18$ boys under 6 feet tall.

41. C. Let:

$$x = \text{length of equal sides in feet}$$
$$x + 8 = \text{length of base in feet}$$

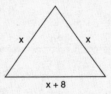

Since the perimeter is 89 feet, the equation is:

$$x + x + (x + 8) = 89$$
$$3x + 8 = 89$$
$$3x + 8 - 8 = 89 - 8$$
$$3x = 81$$
$$\frac{3x}{3} = \frac{81}{3}$$
$$x = 27$$

Hence the length of the base is $x + 8$, or 35 feet.

42. C. Perhaps Joe rounded 90 tiles to 100, and $2.15 to $2.00. This should produce an estimate of about $200, but Joe made a mistake with the decimal point. Two thousand dollars is 10 times as big as $200.

43. A. To solve this equation:

$$\frac{5}{4} = 3y + \frac{1}{4}$$

$$-\frac{1}{4} = \qquad -\frac{1}{4} \qquad\qquad \text{Subtract } \frac{1}{4} \text{ from each side to isolate the variable.}$$

$$1 = 3y \qquad\qquad\qquad \text{And the fraction goes away, too!}$$

$$\frac{1}{3} = \frac{3y}{3} \qquad\qquad\qquad \text{Divide both sides by 3.}$$

$$y = \frac{1}{3}$$

44. A. The shape is formed by two rectangular prisms; to find its volume, find the volume of each prism and add them:

Bottom prism: 8 feet × 10 feet × 2 feet = 160 cubic feet

Top prism: 5 feet × 4 feet × 2 feet = 40 cubic feet

$$160 \text{ cubic feet} + 40 \text{ cubic feet} = 200 \text{ cubic feet}$$

45. B.

$\frac{1}{2}$ of a dollar = \$.50 $\qquad\qquad\qquad\qquad\qquad$ $\frac{3}{4}$ of a dollar = \$.75

$\frac{3}{10}$ of a dollar = \$.30 $\qquad\qquad\qquad\qquad\qquad$ $\frac{3}{20}$ of a dollar = \$.15

$\frac{1}{50}$ of a dollar = \$.02 $\qquad\qquad$ \$.50 + \$.75 + \$.30 + \$.15 + \$.02 = \$1.72

46. B. Since the area of the trapezoid $= \frac{1}{2} \cdot h \cdot (b_1 + b_2)$, you need to find the altitude, h.

Draw altitudes in the figure as follows:

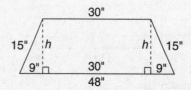

Since the triangles formed are right triangles, you use the Pythagorean theorem, which says:

$$c^2 = a^2 + b^2$$
$$15^2 = 9^2 + h^2$$
$$225 = 81 + h^2$$
$$h^2 = 144$$
$$h = \sqrt{144} = 12 \text{ inches}$$

Hence, the area of the trapezoid will be:

$$\frac{1}{2} \cdot h \cdot (b_1 + b_2) = \frac{1}{2} \cdot 12 \cdot (30 + 48)$$
$$= (6)(78)$$
$$= 468 \text{ square inches}$$

47. A. $75\% = \frac{75}{100} = \frac{3}{4}$. They must win three-fourths of their games to maintain their percentage, so they can lose up to one-fourth of their games. $\frac{1}{4} \times 32 = 8$ games.

48. B. Frequently the relationship expressed first in a verbal description is the operation that must be performed last. In this case, the first relationship to establish is "the product of 10 and n." *Product* means the result of multiplication, which can be expressed as $10n$. One-third of $10n$ can be either expressed as $\frac{10n}{3}$ or $\frac{1}{3}(10n)$. From this quantity, we must then subtract 4. Though choices B and C appear similar, the order of the operations is different, and the result is different. To appreciate this, substitute the value of 1 for n.

$$\frac{10n}{3} - 4 = \frac{10 \cdot 1}{3} - 4 = 3\frac{1}{3} - 4 = -\frac{2}{3}$$

$$\frac{1}{3}(10n - 4) = \frac{1}{3}(10 \cdot 1 - 4) = \frac{1}{3}(6) = 2$$

49. C. Total Area = area of rectangle + $\frac{1}{2}$ area of circle

$$= LW + \frac{1}{2}\pi\left(\frac{W}{2}\right)^2$$

$$= LW + \frac{1}{2}\pi\frac{W^2}{4}$$

$$= LW + \frac{\pi W^2}{8}$$

So the correct answer is Choice C.

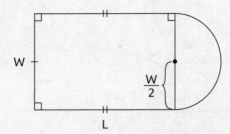

50. C. The y-intercept is the place where the line cuts the y-axis, so the x-coordinate of that point is always 0. For that reason, immediately eliminate choices B, D, and E. Since you are given a slope and a point, you can plug that information into the slope-intercept equation of the line and solve for the y-intercept:

$$y = mx + b$$
$$7 = 1(3) + b$$
$$7 = 3 + 4$$

So the y-intercept is positive 4, and its coordinates are $(0, 4)$.

Answer Sheet for Practice Test 2

(Remove This Sheet and Use It to Mark Your Answers)

1 Ⓐ Ⓑ Ⓒ Ⓓ	26 Ⓐ Ⓑ Ⓒ Ⓓ
2 Ⓐ Ⓑ Ⓒ Ⓓ	27 Ⓐ Ⓑ Ⓒ Ⓓ
3 Ⓐ Ⓑ Ⓒ Ⓓ	28 Ⓐ Ⓑ Ⓒ Ⓓ
4 Ⓐ Ⓑ Ⓒ Ⓓ	29 Ⓐ Ⓑ Ⓒ Ⓓ
5 Ⓐ Ⓑ Ⓒ Ⓓ	30 Ⓐ Ⓑ Ⓒ Ⓓ
6 Ⓐ Ⓑ Ⓒ Ⓓ	31 Ⓐ Ⓑ Ⓒ Ⓓ
7 Ⓐ Ⓑ Ⓒ Ⓓ	32 Ⓐ Ⓑ Ⓒ Ⓓ
8 Ⓐ Ⓑ Ⓒ Ⓓ	33 Ⓐ Ⓑ Ⓒ Ⓓ
9 Ⓐ Ⓑ Ⓒ Ⓓ	34 Ⓐ Ⓑ Ⓒ Ⓓ
10 Ⓐ Ⓑ Ⓒ Ⓓ	35 Ⓐ Ⓑ Ⓒ Ⓓ
11 Ⓐ Ⓑ Ⓒ Ⓓ	36 Ⓐ Ⓑ Ⓒ Ⓓ
12 Ⓐ Ⓑ Ⓒ Ⓓ	37 Ⓐ Ⓑ Ⓒ Ⓓ
13 Ⓐ Ⓑ Ⓒ Ⓓ	38 Ⓐ Ⓑ Ⓒ Ⓓ
14 Ⓐ Ⓑ Ⓒ Ⓓ	39 Ⓐ Ⓑ Ⓒ Ⓓ
15 Ⓐ Ⓑ Ⓒ Ⓓ	40 Ⓐ Ⓑ Ⓒ Ⓓ
16 Ⓐ Ⓑ Ⓒ Ⓓ	41 Ⓐ Ⓑ Ⓒ Ⓓ
17 Ⓐ Ⓑ Ⓒ Ⓓ	42 Ⓐ Ⓑ Ⓒ Ⓓ
18 Ⓐ Ⓑ Ⓒ Ⓓ	43 Ⓐ Ⓑ Ⓒ Ⓓ
19 Ⓐ Ⓑ Ⓒ Ⓓ	44 Ⓐ Ⓑ Ⓒ Ⓓ
20 Ⓐ Ⓑ Ⓒ Ⓓ	45 Ⓐ Ⓑ Ⓒ Ⓓ
21 Ⓐ Ⓑ Ⓒ Ⓓ	46 Ⓐ Ⓑ Ⓒ Ⓓ
22 Ⓐ Ⓑ Ⓒ Ⓓ	47 Ⓐ Ⓑ Ⓒ Ⓓ
23 Ⓐ Ⓑ Ⓒ Ⓓ	48 Ⓐ Ⓑ Ⓒ Ⓓ
24 Ⓐ Ⓑ Ⓒ Ⓓ	49 Ⓐ Ⓑ Ⓒ Ⓓ
25 Ⓐ Ⓑ Ⓒ Ⓓ	50 Ⓐ Ⓑ Ⓒ Ⓓ

CUT HERE

Geometry Reference Formulas

CUT HERE

Rectangle

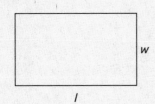

Area = lw
Perimeter = $2l + 2w$

Triangle

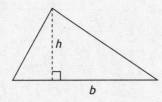

Area = $\frac{1}{2} bh$

Circle

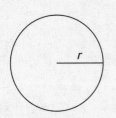

Area = πr^2
Circumference = $2\pi r$

Rectangular Solid

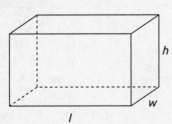

Volume = lwh

Right Circular Cylinder

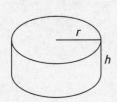

Volume = $\pi r^2 h$

Pythagorean Theorem

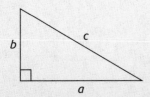

$c^2 = a^2 + b^2$

149

Practice Test 2

90 Minutes

50 Questions

Directions: Solve for each of the following problems. You may use the blank space for scratchwork.

Notes: (1) Unless otherwise specified, the denominators of algebraic expressions appearing in these problems are assumed to be nonzero. (2) Figures that accompany problems are drawn as accurately as possible EXCEPT when it is stated that a figure is not drawn to scale. (3) The Geometry Reference Formulas appearing on the previous page will be printed inside the front cover of the ELM test book.

1. $(2a^2b)^2(3ab^5) =$

   A. $6a^3b^6$
   B. $12ab^5$
   C. $12a^5b^7$
   D. $36a^6b^{12}$
   E. $38a^7b^8$

Teacher	Ticket Sales
Mr. Navarete	480 tickets
Ms. Green	650 tickets
Ms. Schuman	520 tickets
Ms. Petrie	290 tickets
Mr. Frankl	610 tickets
Mr. Peters	140 tickets

2. The sixth grade is having a raffle ticket sale to raise money. The table above shows sales figures for the five classes:

   What is the median number of tickets sold?

   A. 405
   B. 480
   C. 485
   D. 490
   E. 500

3. If the radius of a circle is doubled, then the area of the circle is

   A. doubled
   B. tripled
   C. quadrupled
   D. multiplied times 5
   E. multiplied times $\frac{1}{2}$

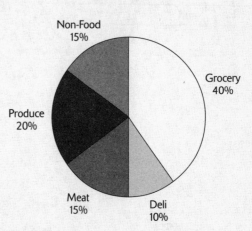

QuickShop Sales

Non-Food 15%
Grocery 40%
Produce 20%
Meat 15%
Deli 10%

4. The graph above shows sales data for QuickShop Market.

   If sales figures for grocery items were $590,000, which of the following figures is the best approximation for produce sales?

   A. $20,000
   B. $300,000
   C. $600,000
   D. $1,200,000
   E. $1,500,000

5. One factor of $8x^2 - 18$ is

A. $8x - 18$

B. $4x - 9$

C. $4x + 9$

D. $8x - 2$

E. $2x + 3$

6. The fraction $\frac{1}{8}$ is between the numbers listed in which of the following pairs?

A. $\frac{1}{10}$ and $\frac{2}{17}$

B. .1 and .12

C. .08 and .1

D. 1 and 2

E. $\frac{1}{9}$ and $\frac{2}{15}$

7. Erin is shopping for blank floppy disks for her computer. A package of 20 brand E disks costs $4.25, while a package of 20 brand Q disks costs $5.75. By purchasing a container of brand E disks, what percent of the cost of brand Q disks will Erin save?

A. 6.5%

B. 26%

C. 35%

D. 150%

E. 156%

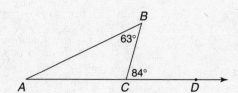

8. Given $\triangle ABC$ with $\angle BCD = 84°$ and $\angle B = 63°$, what is the measure of $\angle A$?

A. 21°

B. 27°

C. 84°

D. 96°

E. 116°

9. $9 + 2x < 4(3 - x)$ is equivalent to

A. $x < -\dfrac{7}{2}$

B. $x > -\dfrac{3}{2}$

C. $x < \dfrac{1}{2}$

D. $x < \dfrac{7}{2}$

E. $x < \dfrac{9}{2}$

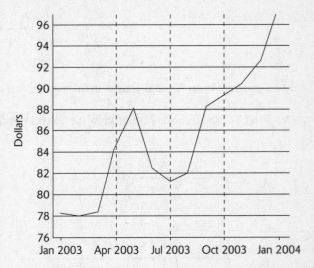

11. The graph above shows the trading price of a particular stock throughout a year, with the value on the *y*-axis representing the price of 1 share of stock.

If Beatrice buys 100 shares at the price shown for February and sells them at the price shown for November, how much money does she make?

A. $12

B. $120

C. $1,200

D. $12,000

E. $120,000

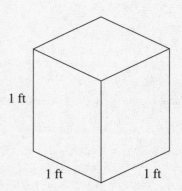

10. The surface area of the cube above is 6 square feet.

If the length of each edge is increased from 1 foot to 3 feet, what is the resulting change in surface area?

A. The surface area would be 3 times as great.

B. The surface area would be 6 times as great.

C. The surface area would be 9 times as great.

D. The surface area would be 27 times as great.

E. The surface area would be 81 times as great.

GO ON TO THE NEXT PAGE

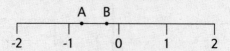

12. Consider Points A and B shown on the number line above.

Which of the following could show the correct position of Point Z, which is the product of A and B?

A.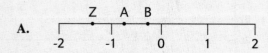

B.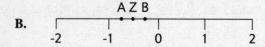

C.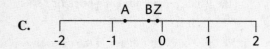

D.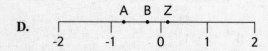

E.

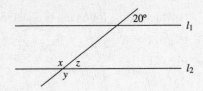

13. In the figure above, l_1 is parallel to l_2. What is the value of $x + y$?

    A. $40°$

    B. $120°$

    C. $160°$

    D. $180°$

    E. $320°$

14. If $\sqrt{x+2} = 3$, then $x =$

    A.   1

    B.   3

    C.   4

    D.   6

    E.   7

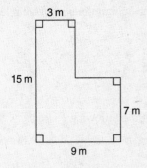

15. What is the perimeter, in meters, of the figure above?

    A.   40

    B.   42

    C.   48

    D.   58

    E.   60

16. $\left(2 - \dfrac{1}{x}\right)\left(\dfrac{x^2}{4x^2 - 1}\right) =$

    A. $\dfrac{x^2}{2x+1}$

    B. $\dfrac{2x}{2x-1}$

    C. $\dfrac{2x}{4x^2-1}$

    D. $\dfrac{x}{2x-1}$

    E. $\dfrac{x}{2x+1}$

GO ON TO THE NEXT PAGE

17. What is the circumference of a circle whose area is 9π?

  A. 18π
  B. 9π
  C. 6π
  D. 9
  E. 6

19. If $x > 0$, which of the following is equal to $\sqrt{72x^5}$?

  A. $36\sqrt{2x^5}$
  B. $36x\sqrt{2x}$
  C. $18x^2\sqrt{2x}$
  D. $6x^2\sqrt{2x}$
  E. $6x\sqrt{2x^2}$

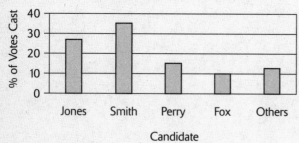

Wisconsin Presidential Primary

18. The graph above shows the result of a recent election.

Which of the following statements about the data is correct?

  A. Jones got more than 30% of the votes.
  B. Smith got twice as many votes as Jones.
  C. The Others combined to get less than 10% of the votes.
  D. Fox got less than a third as many votes as Smith got.
  E. Perry got less votes than Fox.

20. Joe drives a total of 20 miles to get to work. He drives 3 miles to get to the freeway in 9 minutes, 16 miles on the freeway in 18 minutes, and the last mile in 3 minutes. What is his average rate of speed for the whole trip?

  A. 40 miles per hour
  B. 45 miles per hour
  C. 50 miles per hour
  D. 60 miles per hour
  E. 65 miles per hour

21. $\dfrac{4(2a)^2}{8a} =$

   A. a

   B. $2a$

   C. 2

   D. $8a$

   E. 8

22. It takes 6 men 18 hours to do a job. At the same rate, how many men are needed to complete the job in 3 hours?

   A.   1

   B.   12

   C.   21

   D.   30

   E.   36

23. $2\left(x - \dfrac{1}{3}\right) \geq \dfrac{1}{3}$ is equivalent to

   A. $x \geq -\dfrac{1}{3}$

   B. $x \geq \dfrac{1}{4}$

   C. $x \geq \dfrac{1}{2}$

   D. $x \geq 2$

   E. $x \geq 3$

24. The speed limit on many American freeways is 65 miles per hour. About how many kilometers per hour is that? (1 mile = 1.6 kilometers)

   A.   41 kilometers per hour

   B.   67 kilometers per hour

   C.   85 kilometers per hour

   D.   104 kilometers per hour

   E.   110 kilometers per hour

Practice Test 2

GO ON TO THE NEXT PAGE

25. Tom has an average (mean) of 80% for six history tests. His average for the first three of those tests was 72%. He scored 90% on his fourth test, and 88% on his fifth test. What was his score on the sixth test?

    A. 70%

    B. 76%

    C. 80%

    D. 83%

    E. 86%

26. What number is equivalent to $(4)^{-1}(2)^4\left(\frac{1}{2}\right)^2$?

    A. −32

    B. −16

    C. 1

    D. 4

    E. 8

27. Ellen can get to Bill's house by driving 8 miles north, then 6 miles west. Tomorrow is Bill's birthday, and Ellen plans to send a birthday greeting by way of a messenger pigeon, as shown on the map above.

If the messenger pigeon flies directly from Ellen's house to Bill's house, how many miles will the messenger pigeon fly?

    A. 7

    B. 8

    C. 9

    D. 10

    E. 12

28. An $80 jacket is on sale for 40% off. With a coupon, John saves an additional 15% off the reduced price. How much does John save off the original price of the jacket?

    A. $36.00

    B. $39.20

    C. $40.80

    D. $44.00

    E. $45.00

29. What is the total surface area in square meters of a rectangular solid whose length is 7 meters, width is 6 meters, and depth is 3 meters?

    A.   32 square meters
    B.   81 square meters
    C.   126 square meters
    D.   162 square meters
    E.   252 square meters

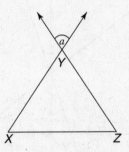

30. In $\triangle XYZ$, $XY = 10$, $YZ = 10$, and $\angle a = 84°$. What is the degree measure of $\angle Z$?

    A.   96°
    B.   84°
    C.   48°
    D.   42°
    E.   24°

31. By halftime the Wolverines had scored 49 points, 18 by their center. Approximately what percent of the team's points were scored by other players?

    A.   17%
    B.   37%
    C.   63%
    D.   83%
    E.   90%

GO ON TO THE NEXT PAGE

32. Which graph represents the solution to the
following system of equations?

$$\begin{cases} -x + y = 3 \\ -4x + 2y = 6 \end{cases}$$

A.

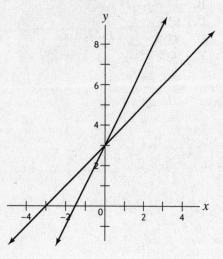

B.

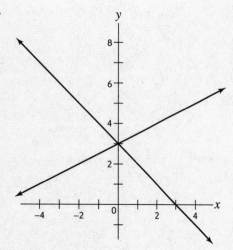

C.

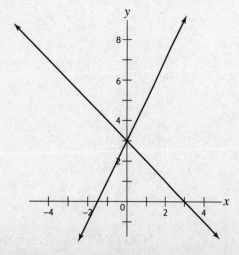

D.

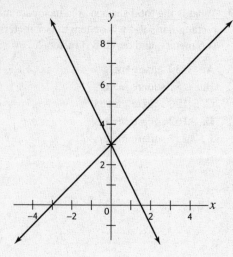

E.

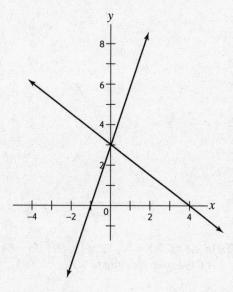

33. $\dfrac{x^2 + 2x}{2} + \dfrac{1}{2x} =$

A. $5x^5 + 1$

B. $\dfrac{x^2 + 2x + 1}{2x}$

C. $\dfrac{x^3 + 2x^2}{2x}$

D. $x^3 + 1$

E. $\dfrac{x^3 + 2x^2 + 1}{2x}$

**Floor space in the Freeman House
(2,000 sq. ft. total)**

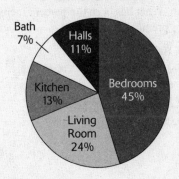

35. Consider the graph above.

How many square feet of floor space are in the Freemans' bathrooms?

A. 7 square feet
B. 70 square feet
C. 140 square feet
D. 1,400 square feet
E. 1,700 square feet

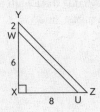

34. In the right triangle XYZ above, $YZ \parallel WU$. What is the length of YZ?

A. 10
B. $\sqrt{164}$
C. $\sqrt{184}$
D. 14
E. 18

36. What is the slope of a line that is parallel to the graph of $5x + 10y = 7$?

A. -2
B. $-\dfrac{1}{2}$
C. $\dfrac{1}{2}$
D. 2
E. 3

GO ON TO THE NEXT PAGE

Practice Test 2

37. In 30 years the price of a premium gasoline has increased from about $.25 a gallon to about $2.75 a gallon. What has been the percent increase in the price of premium gasoline?

    A.   100%
    B.   250%
    C.   1,000%
    D.   2,500%
    E.   3,000%

39. A $100 item is being reduced in price by 50%. With a coupon a customer can save an additional 15% from the reduced price. What is the price of the shirt with a coupon?

    A. $35.00
    B. $42.50
    C. $50.00
    D. $65.00
    E. $70.00

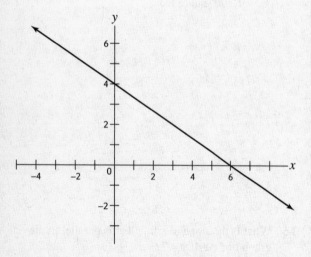

40. If the lengths of two sides of a right triangle are 10 and 11, then what is the length of the third side, which is the longest side?

    A.   10
    B.   11
    C. $\sqrt{120}$
    D. $10\sqrt{2}$
    E. $\sqrt{221}$

38. What is the slope of the line shown in the graph above?

    A. $-\dfrac{3}{2}$

    B. $-\dfrac{2}{3}$

    C. $\dfrac{2}{3}$

    D. $\dfrac{3}{2}$

    E. -4

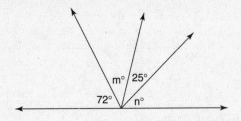

41. In the figure, what is the number of degrees in the sum of $m + n$?

    A.   83

    B.   93

    C.   97

    D.   103

    E.   108

42. Which equation is equivalent to $\frac{1}{2}(4x - 12) - \frac{1}{3}(12 - 3x) = 5$?

    A. $-x - 2 = 5$

    B. $-x - 10 = 5$

    C. $3x - 2 = 5$

    D. $3x - 10 = 0$

    E. $3x - 10 = 5$

43. If $x = \frac{2}{3}$ and $y = -3$, then $xy(10 - y) =$

    A. -26

    B. -14

    C.   14

    D.   26

    E.   28

44. Which equation represents the statement, "The sum of five and y is seven more than x"?

    A. $y = 2 + x$

    B. $2 + y = x$

    C. $5 + x = 7 + y$

    D. $y = 2 + x$

    E. $y + 2 = x$

GO ON TO THE NEXT PAGE

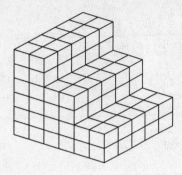

45. The shape above is made from 1-inch cubes. What is the total volume of the shape?

    A.   20 cubic inches

    B.   84 cubic inches

    C.   120 cubic inches

    D.   180 cubic inches

    E.   196 cubic inches

46. A painter paints one-third of a room. The next day he paints one-third of the rest of the room. What fraction of the room still needs to be painted?

    A. $\dfrac{1}{9}$

    B. $\dfrac{1}{3}$

    C. $\dfrac{4}{9}$

    D. $\dfrac{1}{2}$

    E. $\dfrac{5}{9}$

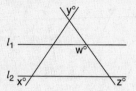

47. If $l_1 \parallel l_2$, $x = 60$, and $w = 2z$, then $y + z =$

    A.   60°

    B.   90°

    C.   120°

    D.   180°

    E.   210°

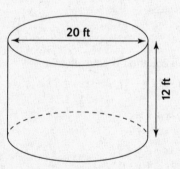

48. The diagram above shows the dimensions of a cylindrical space module.

Which of the following is the best estimate of the maximum volume (in cubic feet) of air the module can hold?

    A.   3,600

    B.   4,500

    C.   7,700

    D.   14,400

    E.   21,200

49. Jennifer is keeping a running total of her purchases at a store to estimate her bill. So far her cart contains:

Item	Price
Books	$34.27
CDs	$12.39
Chicken	$19.75
Computer Printer	$145.99

Which of the following expressions gives the best estimate of Jennifer's checkout bill?

- **A.** 30 + 10 + 20 + 200
- **B.** 30 + 12 + 20 + 100
- **C.** 30 + 10 + 20 + 150
- **D.** 40 + 10 + 20 + 100
- **E.** 40 + 10 + 10 + 200

50. The T table shown in the following figure gives the coordinates of four points on a line. What is the equation of the line?

x	y
0	−1
1	2
2	5
3	8

- **A.** $y = x - 1$
- **B.** $y = 2x$
- **C.** $y = 2x + 1$
- **D.** $y = 3x - 1$
- **E.** $y = 3x + 2$

IF YOU FINISH BEFORE TIME IS CALLED, CHECK YOUR WORK ON THIS SECTION ONLY. DO NOT WORK ON ANY OTHER SECTION IN THE TEST.

Reviewing Practice Test 2

Review your simulated ELM Practice Examination by following these steps:

1. Check the Answer Key that follows. Put a checkmark in the box following any wrong answer.
2. Fill out the Review Chart (page 168).
3. Read all explanations (pages 169–176). Go back to review any explanations that are not clear to you.
4. Fill out the Reasons for Mistakes chart on page 168.
5. Go back to the math review section and review any basic skills necessary before taking the next practice test.

Don't leave out any of these steps. They are very important in learning to do your best on the ELM.

Answer Key for Practice Test 2

(Number Sense – NS) (Algebra – Al) (Geometry – G)

1. C ❑ (Al)
2. E ❑ (NS)
3. C ❑ (G)
4. B ❑ (NS)
5. E ❑ (Al)
6. E ❑ (NS)
7. B ❑ (NS)
8. A ❑ (G)
9. C ❑ (Al)
10. C ❑ (G)
11. C ❑ (NS)
12. D ❑ (NS)
13. E ❑ (G)
14. E ❑ (Al)
15. C ❑ (G)
16. E ❑ (Al)
17. C ❑ (G)
18. D ❑ (NS)
19. D ❑ (Al)
20. A ❑ (NS)
21. B ❑ (Al)
22. E ❑ (NS)
23. C ❑ (Al)
24. D ❑ (NS)
25. E ❑ (NS)

26. C ❑ (Al)
27. D ❑ (G)
28. B ❑ (NS)
29. D ❑ (G)
30. C ❑ (G)
31. C ❑ (NS)
32. A ❑ (Al)
33. E ❑ (Al)
34. D ❑ (G)
35. C ❑ (NS)
36. B ❑ (Al)
37. C ❑ (NS)
38. B ❑ (Al)
39. B ❑ (NS)
40. E ❑ (G)
41. A ❑ (G)
42. E ❑ (Al)
43. A ❑ (Al)
44. D ❑ (Al)
45. C ❑ (G)
46. C ❑ (G)
47. C ❑ (G)
48. A ❑ (G)
49. C ❑ (NS)
50. D ❑ (G)

Review Chart

Use your marked Answer Key to fill in the following chart for the multiple-choice questions.

	Possible	Completed	Right	Wrong
Number Sense (NS)	17			
Algebra (Al)	16			
Geometry (G)	17			
Totals	**50**			

Reasons for Mistakes

Fill out the following chart only after you have read all the explanations that follow. This chart will help you spot your strengths and weaknesses and your repeated errors or trends in types of errors.

	Total Missed	Simple Mistake	Misread Problem	Lack of Knowledge
Number Sense (NS)				
Algebra (Al)				
Geometry (G)				
Totals				

Examine your results carefully. Reviewing the above information will help you pinpoint your common mistakes. Focus on avoiding your most common mistakes as you practice. The "Lack of Knowledge" column will help you focus your review in the math review section. If you are missing a lot of questions because of "Lack of Knowledge," you should go back and spend extra time reviewing the basics.

Answer Explanations for Practice Test 2

1. **C.** The trick is to note that the first term is squared. It might be helpful to rewrite the expression:

$$(2a^2b)^2(3ab^5) = (2a^2b)(2a^2b)(3ab^5) = (2 \times 2 \times 3)(aaaaa)(bbbbbbb) = 12a^5b^7$$

2. **E.** To find the median, first arrange the data values in numerical order:

$$140, 290, 480, 520, 610, 650$$

When there are an even number of data values, the median is the mean of the middle two values:

$$\frac{480 + 520}{2} = 500$$

3. **C.** Since the area formula of a circle is $A = \pi r^2$, if you double the radius, the area is quadrupled. Try some simple numbers. If $r = 1$, then $A = \pi(1)^2$, so $A = \pi$. If $r = 2$, then $A = \pi(2)^2$, so $A = 4\pi$.

4. **B.** Grocery sales are 40%, and produce sales are 20%—half as much. So, the dollar value of produce sales should be half the value of grocery sales. Since $590,000 is approximately $600,000, and you are being asked for the *best* approximation, use $600,000 for any calculations. Half of $600,000 is $300,000.

5. **E.** First factor out 2, leaving $4x^2 - 9$. Now factor the difference of two squares:

$$4x^2 - 9 = (2x + 3)(2x + 3)$$

So one factor is $2x + 3$.

6. **E.** The fraction $\frac{1}{8}$ equals .125. Thus, it would lie between $\frac{1}{9}$ (.111 . . .) and $\frac{2}{15}$ (.133 . . .).

7. **B.** The cost of a container of Brand Q is $5.75. The cost of a container of Brand E is $4.25. The difference between the two prices is $1.50, which represents a savings of $1.50. Brand Q costs $5.75, so $\frac{\$1.50}{\$5.75} = .2608 = 26.08\%$. The correct answer is Choice B.

8. **A.** $\angle BCD = \angle A + \angle B$ (exterior angle of a triangle equals the sum of the opposite two). Then $84° = \angle A + 63°$ and $\angle A = 21°$

9. **C.** To solve this, you must first expand the expression on the right side, isolate the variable, and then divide by the coefficient:

$$9 + 2x < 4(3 - x)$$
$$9 + 2x < 12 - 4x \qquad \text{Add } 4x \text{ to both sides.}$$
$$9 + 6x < 12 \qquad \text{Subtract 9 from both sides.}$$
$$6x < 3 \qquad \text{Divide both sides by 6.}$$
$$x < \frac{1}{2}$$

10. **C.** The surface area of each face of the original cube is 1 square foot. However, if the edge is increased to 3 feet, the surface area of each face becomes 3 feet × 3 feet, or 9 feet. So the surface area is increased by a factor of 9.

11. **C.** The price shown for February is about $78 per share, so the cost of 100 shares is about $7,800. The price for November is about $90, so the proceeds from the sale of 100 shares are about $9,000. Beatrice's profit is the difference between the proceeds and the cost, which is $1,200. Choices A, B, D, and E aren't even close.

12. D. A and B are negative numbers, so their product has to be positive. Only Choice D shows Z as a positive number.

13. E. If l_1 and l_2 are parallel, then $z = 20°$. If $z = 20°$, $\angle x$ equals 160°, because they form a straight line. Since x and y are vertical, $\angle y$ is also 160°. Therefore, $160° + 160° = 320°$.

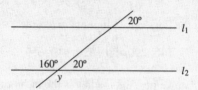

14. E. Squaring both sides gives

$$(\sqrt{x} + 2)^2 = 3^2$$
$$x + 2 = 9$$

Now subtract 2:
$$x = 7$$

You could have worked from the answers by plugging in.

15. C. Notice how drawing some line segments can assist you in finding the necessary lengths.

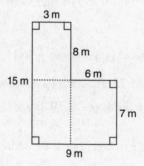

The perimeter is the sum of the lengths of the sides.

$$P = 15 + 3 + 8 + 6 + 7 + 9 = 48 \text{ m}$$

16. E. First simplify the term on the left:

$$\left(2 - \frac{1}{x}\right) = \frac{2x}{x} - \frac{1}{x} = \frac{2x - 1}{x}$$

Next notice that you can factor the denominator in the term on the right:

$$\left(\frac{x^2}{4x^2 - 1}\right) = \frac{x^2}{(2x + 1)(2x - 1)}$$

Now the two terms are as follows:

$$\left(\frac{(2x - 1)}{x}\right)\left(\frac{x^2}{(2x + 1)(2x - 1)}\right)$$

Now cancel as follows:

$$\left(\frac{(2x - 1)^1}{x}\right)\left(\frac{x^{2^1}}{(2x + 1)(2x - 1)^1}\right)$$

Leaves

$$\frac{x}{2x + 1}$$

17. C. Since the formula for the area of a circle is $A = \pi r^2$, and the circumference formula is $C = 2\pi r$, first use the area formula to solve for the radius.

$$A = \pi r^2$$
$$9\pi = \pi r^2$$
$$\frac{9\pi}{\pi} = \frac{\pi r^2}{\pi}$$
$$9 = r^2$$
$$3 = r$$

Now plug the radius of 3 into the circumference formula:

$$C = 2\pi r$$
$$C = 2\pi(3)$$
$$C = 6\pi$$

18. D. Statement A is false; Jones got *less* than 30%. Statements B and C area also false. Statement D is true: Fox got 10%, whereas Smith got about 35%. Ten percent is less than a third of 35%.

19. D. Simplify the problem as follows: $\sqrt{72x^5} = \sqrt{36 \cdot 2 \cdot x^4 \cdot x}$. Since $\sqrt{36}$ is 6, and $\sqrt{x^4}$ is x^2, then $\sqrt{36 \cdot 2 \cdot x^4 \cdot x} = 6x^2\sqrt{2x}$. You could also work from the answers.

20. A. We are comparing miles to time, either minutes or hours. Since the information is given in minutes, it's best to start with minutes:

$$\frac{3 + 16 + 1}{9 + 18 + 3} = \frac{20}{30} = \frac{2}{3}$$

So, Joe drives 2 miles in every 3 minutes. Or, Joe drives $\frac{2}{3}$ of a mile per minute. Since the answer choices are given in terms of miles per hour, we'd better convert this to miles per hour to be sure it is incorrect.

$$\frac{2}{3} \times \frac{20}{20} = \frac{40}{60} = 40 \text{ miles for } 60 \text{ minutes, or } 40 \text{ miles per hour}$$

21. B. To simplify this expression:

$$\frac{4(2a)^2}{8a}$$

First, square the quantity in parentheses:

$$\frac{4(4a^2)}{8a}$$

Then, multiply the factors in the numerator:

$$\frac{16a^2}{8a}$$

Then, divide the numerator by the denominator:

$$\frac{16a^2}{8a} = \frac{16}{8} \cdot \frac{a^2}{a} = 2a$$

22. E. Three hours is one-sixth as long as 18 hours. To do the job in one-sixth of the time, six times as many workers are needed.

$$6 \times 6 \text{ workers} = 36 \text{ workers}$$

23. C. To solve this inequality:

$$2\left(x - \frac{1}{3}\right) \geq \frac{1}{3}$$

$$2x - \frac{2}{3} \geq \frac{1}{3} \qquad \text{Expand the left side of the inequality.}$$

$$\underline{+\frac{2}{3} \quad +\frac{2}{3}} \qquad \text{Add } \frac{2}{3} \text{ to both sides to isolate the variable.}$$

$$2x \geq 1$$

$$x \geq \frac{1}{2} \qquad \text{Divide both sides by 2.}$$

24. D. To solve this problem, multiply 65 by 1.6, or estimate. The result is a number that is a little more than one-and-a-half times as large as 65. The only reasonable answer is Choice D.

25. E. Since Tom had a mean of 80% after six tests, he must have had a total of 480 points because $480 \div 6 = 80$. Tom's average after three tests was 72%, so after three tests he had 216 points because $3 \times 72 = 216$. When his fourth and fifth tests are added to this, the result is 394. So his sixth test had to be the difference between the total points he needed (480) and the points he had after five tests (394). $480 - 394 = 86$.

26. C. Rewriting this might help to simplify it. The base gives the factor, the exponent tells how many times to use it as a factor. A positive number raised to a negative exponent becomes a fraction, not a negative number.

$$(4)^{-1}(2)^4\left(\frac{1}{2}\right)^2 = \left(\frac{1}{4}\right)(2 \cdot 2 \cdot 2 \cdot 2)\left(\frac{1}{2} \cdot \frac{1}{2}\right) = \frac{1}{4} \cdot 16 \cdot \frac{1}{4} = \frac{16}{16} = 1$$

27. D. To find the third side of this right triangle, use the Pythagorean theorem:

$$a^2 + b^2 = c^2$$
$$8^2 + 6^2 = c^2$$
$$64 + 36 = c^2$$
$$100 = c^2$$
$$10 = c \text{ (because } 10 \times 10 = 100)$$

b = 6 miles

c = 10 miles

a = 8 miles

28. B. Forty percent of 80 is $32. John saves 15% of the reduced price. The reduced price is $80 - $32 = $48. Fifteen percent of $48 is $7.20. So, John saves $32 + $7.20 = $39.20.

29. D. A rectangle solid consists of six rectangular faces. This one in particular has two 7×6, two 6×3, and two 7×3 rectangles with areas of 42, 18, and 12, respectively. Therefore, the total surface area will be:

$$2(42) + 2(18) + 2(21) = 84 + 36 + 42 = 162 \text{ square meters}$$

30. C. Since $XY = YZ = 10$, $\triangle XYZ$ is an isosceles triangle and $\angle X = \angle Z$. $\angle Y = 84°$ because it forms a vertical angle with the given angle.

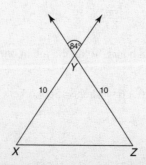

$$\angle X + \angle Y + \angle Z = 180°$$
$$\angle X + 84° + \angle Z = 180°$$
$$2(\angle Z) + 84° = 180°$$
$$2(\angle Z) = 96°$$
$$\angle Z = 48°$$

31. C. The rest of the team scored $49 - 18 = 31$ points, so we can set up a proportion to solve the problem:

$$\frac{31}{49} = \frac{x}{100}$$

Since 49 is close to half of 100, to estimate, just double 31; so 31 is close to 62% of 49. The only answer close to that is C.

32. A. The answer is the graph that represents these two equations. The easiest way to determine that is to convert these two equations to the slope-intercept form, $y = mx + b$.

$$-x + y = 3 \rightarrow y = x + 3$$
$$-4x + 2y = 6 \rightarrow y = 2x + 3$$

The lines in the answer both have a positive slope and y-intercept of $+3$. Lines with a positive slope travel upward from left to right; the y-intercept is the point on the y-axis that the line passes through. All four answers show graphs with correct y-intercepts. However, only Graph A shows two lines with a positive slope, so we can identify it as the only possible answer without going any further.

33. E. Since the common denominator is $2x$, simply multiply the first term by x, then add the numerators and keep the denominator.

$$\frac{x^2 + 2x}{2} + \frac{1}{2x}$$

$$\frac{(x)(x^2 + 2x)}{(x)2} + \frac{1}{2x}$$

$$\frac{x^3 + 2x^2}{2x} + \frac{1}{2x} = \frac{x^3 + 2x^2 + 1}{2x}$$

34. D. Since $YZ \parallel WU$, then $UZ = 2$. So $XY = 8$ and $XZ = 10$.

Plug into the Pythagorean theorem as follows:

$$a^2 + b^2 = c^2$$
$$(8)^2 + (10)^2 = c^2$$
$$64 + 100 = c^2$$
$$164 = c^2$$
$$\sqrt{164} = c$$

35. C. The bathrooms are 7% of 2,000 square feet. Seven percent of 200 is 14. Seven percent of 2,000 is 10 times as much, which is 140 square feet.

36. B. Lines that are parallel have the same slope. The difficulty is that, in this problem, the equation of a line is given in the standard form, not the slope-intercept form (which is $y = mx + b$), where m, the coefficient of x, is the slope of the line. The easiest way to get the slope is to just rework the equation into the slope-intercept form:

$$5x + 10y = 7$$
$$10y = -5x + 7$$
$$y = -\frac{1}{2}x + \frac{7}{10}$$

So the slope is $-\frac{1}{2}$, which is Choice B.

37. C. When calculating percent change, use the formula:

$$\frac{\text{change in price}}{\text{starting price}} = \frac{\text{percent}}{100}$$

The change in price = \$2.75 – \$.25 = \$2.50; the starting price = \$.25, so:

$$\frac{\$2.50}{\$.25} = \frac{x}{100}$$

To solve a proportion, you can cross-multiply and set the products equal:

$$\$250 = \$.25x$$

Then:

$$\frac{\$250}{\$.25} = \frac{\$.25x}{\$.25}$$

$$x = 1,000$$

38. B. Since the line slopes downward from left to right, it has a negative slope—therefore you can eliminate choices C and D. Slope is defined as:

$$\frac{vertical\ shift}{horizontal\ shift}$$

In this case, the line goes down two units for every three units it moves to the right:

$$\frac{-2}{3} = -\frac{2}{3}$$

39. B. One hundred dollars reduced by 50% leaves a price of \$50. Fifty dollars reduced by 15% is a reduction of \$7.50; \$50 – \$7.50 = \$42.50.

40. E. Plug into the Pythagorean theorem as follows:

$$a^2 + b^2 = c^2$$
$$(10)^2 + (11)^2 = c^2$$
$$100 + 121 = c^2$$
$$221 = c^2$$
$$\sqrt{221} = c$$

41. A. Since the sum of the angles is 180°, we have:

$$m + n + 72 + 25 = 180$$
$$m + n + 97 = 180$$
$$m + n = 180 - 97$$
$$m + n \text{ is } 83°$$

Hence, the sum of $m + n$ is 83°.

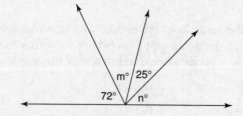

42. E. To simplify the left side of the equation, you must distribute the multiplication by each factor outside the parentheses to the terms within the parentheses, then combine like terms:

$$\frac{1}{2}(4x-12)-\frac{1}{3}(12-3x)=5$$

$$\left(\frac{1}{2}\right)(4x)-\left(\frac{1}{2}\right)(12)+\left(-\frac{1}{3}\right)(12)+\left(-\frac{1}{3}\right)(-3x)=5$$

$$2x-6-4+x=5$$

$$3x-10=5$$

43. A. To evaluate this expression, plug the given values in for the variables, and perform the operations:

$$xy(10-y)=\left(\frac{2}{3}\right)(-3)(10-[-3])=(-2)(13)=-26$$

44. D. The "sum of five and y" is $5 + y$. "Seven more than x" is $7 + x$. Because they are equal, we can say that $5 + y = 7 + x$. However, that answer choice is not available. By subtracting five from each side, we can simplify the relationship.

$$y = 2 + x$$

45. C. You cannot use a simple formula for calculating the volume of the shape because it is not a prism. However, with a little manipulation, you can create a prism that has an equivalent volume:

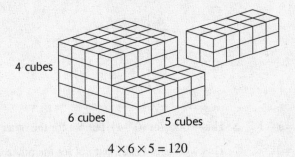

$$4 \times 6 \times 5 = 120$$

46. C. On day one, the painter paints one-third of the room; so he *doesn't* paint two-thirds of the room. The next day he paints one-third of the *rest* of the room—so he paints one-third of the two-thirds—so he *doesn't* paint two-thirds of two-thirds. $\frac{2}{3} \times \frac{2}{3} = \frac{4}{9}$

47. C. Because $l_1 \parallel l_2$, the corresponding angles formed on lines l_1 and l_2 are equal:

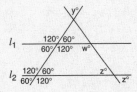

In any quadrilateral, the sum of interior degrees equals $360°$. Therefore, $\angle w + \angle z = 180°$. If $w = 2z$, $\angle w = 120°$, and $\angle z = 60°$. Therefore:

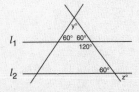

$\angle y = 60°$ (because there are $180°$ in a triangle). So the sum of $y + z = 60° + 60° = 120°$.

175

48. A. To find the volume of a container that stands up straight with its sides perpendicular to its base:

First find the area (A) of its base (a circle):

$$\pi \times (\text{radius})^2 \qquad [A = \pi r^2]$$

Then, multiply this number by the container's height. So,

$$\text{Volume} = \pi \times (\text{radius})^2 \times \text{height} = 3.14(10)^2(12)$$
$$= 3.14(100)(12), \text{ or approximately } 3(100)(12) = 3,600$$

Reminder: The term *radius* refers to the distance from the center of the circle to the circle's edge (halfway across), and the formula for finding the area (A) of a circle is

$$A = \pi r^2$$

Pi, or π, is approximately 3.14.

49. C. The expression for this answer rounds each item to the closest $10. Choices B and C round the computer printer to the closest $100, which introduces a significant error of about $46. Choice A incorrectly rounds the printer to $200, introducing an even bigger error.

50. D. If you aren't familiar with techniques for solving this problem, the easiest way is to substitute x and y values from the table in the answer choices to see which equation works with all the x and y pairs.

x	y
0	−1
1	2
2	5
3	8

$y = x - 1$ This works for (0, −1), but not for the other values.

$y = 2x$ This works for (1, 2), but not for the other values.

$y = 2x + 1$ This works for (2, 5), but not for the other values.

$y = 3x - 1$ This works for all given (x, y) pairs.

PART IV

ANALYSIS OF THE EPT EXAM AREAS

Introduction to the English Placement Test (EPT)

The purpose of the English Placement Test is to determine whether you are prepared to undertake college-level work in reading and writing. The results of the test will be used to place you in the appropriate course.

The EPT is composed of three sections and is 1 hour and 45 minutes long. The three sections and the timing for those sections are as follows:

Essay	1 Question	45 Minutes
Reading Skills	45 Multiple-Choice Questions	30 Minutes
Composing Skills	45 Multiple-Choice Questions	30 Minutes

The sections above will be carefully reviewed in the following pages. A complete simulated practice test is also included. You may have a sample EPT diagnosed online through the testing service.

The English Placement Test Online

You can have your reading, composing, and essay writing skills diagnosed through the CSU/EPT Diagnostic Writing Service (DWS). To reach this service, go online at **http://www.essayeval.org.**

For the reading and composing skills sections of the test, you may take a free, self-correcting practice exam that is made up of questions from previous EPT statewide exams. Once you submit the test, it is scored instantly and you are provided with explanations of any questions you miss.

For the essay portion of the test, you can have your writing diagnosed by CSU faculty for a small fee. Through this service, individual students or entire classes of students can submit essays responding to EPT essay questions and have their essays read by CSU faculty. Within 10 business days, you should receive your essays back online, with diagnostic comments. DWS is also available as a paper-and-pencil service. Students using the paper service must wait about 3 to 4 weeks to receive their reader feedback.

Scoring the EPT

The "cut score" for the EPT is 151 on a scale that goes from 120 to 180 (lowest–highest). If you score at or above the cut score, you will be placed in regular, college-level English classes. If you score below 151, you will need to take remedial coursework in English. Scores for the component parts of the EPT are also given—Reading Skills (120–180), Composing Skills (120–180), and the Essay (1–6).

Introduction to the Essay Section

The EPT essay is based on a short quotation or passage. The time given to plan and write the essay is 45 minutes.

Essay Score

Each essay is read independently and scored holistically by two faculty members who use a scoring guide that defines levels of performance on the essay. The two readers' scores are totaled to give the student's reported essay score, which falls between scores of 2 (low) and 12 (high)—the scoring guidelines are outlined in a later section.

Students must write on the assigned topic, demonstrate an understanding of the reading passage, and support their generalizations with specific reasons and examples. Such matters as clarity of thought, fluency, careful organization, development of ideas, and the use of clear and precise language all have an important influence upon the score given by each reader.

A different topic is used each time the test is given; all students taking the test at the same time write on the same topic. Topics are designed to allow all students to display their best writing. The topics selected are of general interest and should be accessible to all groups of EPT candidates. All essay topics are pretested at CSU campuses and are given final approval by the English Placement Test Development Committee.

The Diagnostic Writing Service Comments

The comprehensive DWS comments (if you use the diagnostic writing service) provide specific diagnostic help to the students and to their teachers. Specifically, the DWS comments explain to students:

- how fully and effectively they have responded to the essay task
- how well they have developed and supported their argument
- how well-chosen their examples are
- how sound their reasoning is
- how well they have organized and connected their ideas
- how well they have maintained control of sentences, of diction, and of syntax
- how well they have shown command of standard written English

CSU English Placement Test Scoring Guide

At each of the six score points for on-topic papers, descriptors of writing performance are lettered so that:

a. = response to the topic

b. = understanding and use of the passage

c. = quality and clarity of thought

d. = organization, development, and support

e. = syntax and command of language

f. = grammar, usage, and mechanics

Score of 6: Superior

A **6** essay is superior writing, but may have minor flaws.

A typical essay in this category:

a. addresses the topic clearly and responds effectively to all aspects of the task

b. demonstrates a thorough critical understanding of the passage in developing an insightful response

c. explores the issues thoughtfully and in depth

d. is coherently organized and developed, with ideas supported by apt reasons and well-chosen examples

e. has an effective, fluent style marked by syntactic variety and a clear command of language

f. is generally free from errors in grammar, usage, and mechanics

Score of 5: Strong

A **5** essay demonstrates clear competence in writing. It may have some errors, but they are not serious enough to distract or confuse the reader.

A typical essay in this category:

a. addresses the topic clearly, but may respond to some aspects of the task more effectively than others

b. demonstrates a sound critical understanding of the passage in developing a well-reasoned response

c. shows some depth and complexity of thought

d. is well organized and developed, with ideas supported by appropriate reasons and examples

e. displays some syntactic variety and facility in the use of language

f. may have a few errors in grammar, usage, and mechanics

Score of 4: Adequate

A **4** essay demonstrates adequate writing. It may have some errors that distract the reader, but they do not significantly obscure meaning.

A typical essay in this category:

a. addresses the topic, but may slight some aspects of the task

b. demonstrates a generally accurate understanding of the passage in developing a sensible response

c. may treat the topic simplistically or repetitively

d. is adequately organized and developed, generally supporting ideas with reasons and examples

e. demonstrates adequate use of syntax and language

f. may have some errors, but generally demonstrates control of grammar, usage, and mechanics

Score of 3: Marginal

A **3** essay demonstrates developing competence, but is flawed in some significant way(s).

A typical essay in this category reveals *one or more* of the following weaknesses:

a. distorts or neglects aspects of the task

b. demonstrates some understanding of the passage, but may misconstrue parts of it or make limited use of it in developing a weak response

c. lacks focus, or demonstrates confused or simplistic thinking

d. is poorly organized and developed, presenting generalizations without adequate and appropriate support or presenting details without generalizations

e. has limited control of syntax and vocabulary

f. has an accumulation of errors in grammar, usage, and mechanics that sometimes interfere with meaning

Score of 2: Very Weak

A **2** essay is seriously flawed.

A typical essay in this category reveals *one or more* of the following weaknesses:

a. indicates confusion about the topic or neglects important aspects of the task

b. demonstrates very poor understanding of the main points of the passage, does not use the passage appropriately in developing a response, or may not use the passage at all

    c. lacks focus and coherence, and often fails to communicate its ideas

    d. has very weak organization and development, providing simplistic generalizations without support

    e. has inadequate control of syntax and vocabulary

    f. is marred by numerous errors in grammar, usage, and mechanics that frequently interfere with meaning

Score of 1: Incompetent

A **1** essay demonstrates fundamental deficiencies in writing skills.

A typical essay in this category reveals *one or more* of the following weaknesses:

    a. suggests an inability to comprehend the question or to respond meaningfully to the topic

    b. demonstrates little or no ability to understand the passage or to use it in developing a response

    c. is unfocused, illogical, or incoherent

    d. is disorganized and undeveloped, providing little or no relevant support

    e. lacks basic control of syntax and vocabulary

    f. has serious and persistent errors in grammar, usage, and mechanics that severely interfere with meaning

Readers should not penalize ESL writers excessively for slight shifts in idiom, problems with articles, confusion over prepositions, and *occasional* misuse of verb tense and verb forms, so long as such features do not obscure meaning.

A Close Look at the Essay

There are a number of ways to approach writing an in-class type essay. If you've been practicing for this part of the exam in your English class, and you and your teacher are satisfied with the way you handle these types of essays, you can skim this section focusing on the type of writing task and continue to write your essays your way. If you aren't confident with your technique or wish to review the process with a few successful techniques, then read this section carefully.

Reviewing the Writing Process

For any writing task, you should envision three steps leading to the finished product:

1. Preparing to write (Pre-writing)
2. Writing
3. Proofreading (Editing)

Preparing to Write (Pre-writing)

Read the topic and the assignment carefully. Circle or underline key words to help you focus on the assigned task. Reread the assignment. If there are several tasks given, number them and write them down. Let the nature of the assignment determine the structure of your essay. **Notice that this essay question gives you two tasks: (1) it requires that you explain the argument given, and (2) it asks you take a position either agreeing or disagreeing with the argument (including specific supporting details).**

Regardless of the structure of the essay, take time to organize your thoughts on paper before writing. The three basic techniques are brainstorming, clustering, and outlining.

Brainstorming is simply jotting down in the scratch area provided as many general thoughts and specific ideas that might help you analyze the argument and take a position on whether you agree or disagree. You may wish to make a simple list or chart. Neatness, order, and spelling do not matter at this point.

Clustering provides a way to put all of your thoughts down on paper before you write so that you can quickly see the structure of the whole paper. As you analyze the argument and take a position, you may write down some information in the pre-writing area and draw a circle around the key word or words in your analysis and then draw a circle around the position you are taking. Then think of all the specific elements you might use and connect them to the central topic clusters.

You can then number the parts of the cluster (the elements) to give an order to your thoughts. You don't have to use all the elements of your cluster.

Outlining, although mentioned last here, is a well-known, outstanding technique. Keeping your outline simple will make it easier to use. The basic structure of the type of outline you should use is:

<u>**Introduction**</u>

<u>**Body or Discussion**</u>

<u>**Conclusion**</u>

Using this structure will help you build an organized essay.

Remember, spend at least 4 or 5 minutes pre-writing and organizing your ideas before you start writing.

Writing the Essay

Opening Paragraph

A strong opening paragraph is essential for a well-developed response. One method is to explain the argument in the first paragraph and then further show an understanding of the argument and take a stand in the second paragraph. Another method is to explain the argument and give an indication of whether you agree or disagree, all in the first paragraph. In explaining the argument, it is entirely appropriate and often desirable to use short quotations from the argument (in quotation marks). However, be sure not to quote long parts of the passage. Instead, choose short pieces that you combine smoothly with your own words.

An effective first paragraph will keep you focused on the tasks given. Remember, you will typically be asked to explain the argument and either agree or disagree using specific supporting details. Note that you might agree or disagree only in part; that is, you will have points both pro and con, which you will investigate and clarify in the body of the essay.

Body or Discussion

Writing the body of the response involves presenting specific details and examples that relate to the aspects that you will introduce and/or fulfill the requirements of the tasks given. (The second paragraph may start by giving your position on the argument if you haven't done so in the opening paragraph.)

The body may consist of one long paragraph or several shorter paragraphs. If you choose to break your discussion into several paragraphs, make sure that each consists of at least three sentences. Very short paragraphs may make your response appear insubstantial and scattered.

Be realistic about how much you can write. Although the readers want you to support your points adequately, they understand that you must write concisely to finish in time. Providing at least one substantial example, or "for instance," is important for each aspect you discuss in the body of your response.

Conclusion

As you prepare to write the conclusion, you should pay special attention to time. Having a formal conclusion to your response is unnecessary, but a conclusion should function to (1) complete your response to the question and/or (2) add information that you failed to introduce earlier.

Proofreading

Always allow a few minutes to proofread your essay for errors in grammar, usage, and spelling. If you detect an error, simply line it out carefully and neatly insert the correction. Keep in mind, both while you are writing and while you are correcting, that your handwriting should be legible. Even though readers are instructed to ignore the quality of handwriting, if the paper is too difficult to read, they might get a negative impression of the essay.

Sample Topic

Directions: You will have 45 minutes to plan and write an essay on the topic assigned below. Before you begin writing, read the passage carefully and plan what you will say. Your essay should be as well organized and as carefully written as you can make it.

"This country's founders wrote into the constitution of their new nation safeguards for the personal rights of the citizens, most comprehensive of which is the right to life, liberty, and the pursuit of happiness. But there is an ominous corporate trend that threatens these cherished ideals. Many companies have decreed that smoking is banned in the workplace. Their stated reasoning is that smoking is unhealthy, both to the smokers and to those exposed to their second-hand smoke. The underlying reasoning is the belief that smokers cost more than do nonsmokers in health-care claims. But some companies have expanded the smoking ban and threaten to fire employees if they smoke anywhere outside the workplace, including their homes. This trend endangers our personal freedoms. Will corporate America soon follow us home and monitor our Thanksgiving meal so we will not become obese? Will they whip us around the jogging track so that we will maintain the level of fitness they determine we should have?"

—Gladys Schoonover

Explain Schoonover's argument and discuss the extent to which you agree or disagree with her analysis. Support your position, providing reasons and examples from your own experience, observations, or reading.

Student Essay

Ms. Schoonover suggests that corporate America, in banning smoking outside the work area, is overstepping and that this trend is "ominous" and may threaten our right to "life, liberty, and the pursuit of happiness." The question she raises is not whether smoking is bad for a person but whether others have the right to tell individuals how to behave in their personal lives and, in addition, whether it is right for an employer to have such power over their employees. She further suggests, by asking if companies will follow us home to see that we eat properly ("monitor our Thanksgiving meal") or exercise to keep fit ("whip us around the jogging track"), if these restrictions will expand to include other parts of our lives as well.

Schoonover brings up difficult questions. They include how much control a business should have over it's workers in a free society, how much personal freedom can be curtailed and for what reasons by anybody other than the person himself or herself. And these are not questions that have only to do with smoking. They are fundamental concerns about what people can and can't do with their own lives and whether anyone can or should tell them how to behave. And the question involves finally more than just businesses—for example, government, private associations, and so forth. An important point is whether a person's behavior hurts another person. And I feel that it is this that ought to determine whether someone can tell an adult what he or she should do or not do.

I know that many restaurants now ban smoking, which is their right to do inside their own establishments for the protection of their customers from second-hand smoke. Here, the reason behind the ban is so that one person's behavior won't harm another person. But should that restaurant have the right to limit the amount people can eat so they won't get fat? I don't think so. Eating too much isn't harming the other people in the restaurant. Governments ban many things that are considered crimes—murder, arson, robbery, to name just a few—because these actions are harmful to people. These bans are appropriate. And in less important areas, governments ban such things as taking your dog for a walk and leaving his waste behind or having your dog off a leash. This too is sensible because animal waste can breed germs and a loose dog might bite or run in front of a car, causing an accident. But other restrictions can be very questionable. Should a city say, for example, that you can't park your car on the street? They would have to be very careful about a restriction like that and would have to prove that somehow parking your car there would be harmful to others.

I believe that with freedom also comes responsibility. The person who chooses to smoke at home has that right, and the company that person works for does not have the right to fire him because of it. But also the person who smokes at home must take responsibility for not harming others in the home, and it is a matter for the family members to work out among themselves. A person who drinks alcohol has the responsibility to not drink too much and to not drive if they have been drinking. But finally, if you do not harm others by your actions, you have a right to live your life as you choose and it is not the place of anyone to take away that right.

Analysis of the Student Essay

This is a strong essay and would score in the top third of the scale. The writer clearly understands the argument of the topic and explains that understanding quite competently in the first paragraph. The writer also uses quotations from the topic well, paraphrasing often and adding short direct quotations where appropriate. The writer clearly understands that the topic is not restricted to concerns about smoking but includes much wider questions involving personal freedoms in general.

The essay is well organized, with the first paragraph explaining the topic's argument, the second expanding the understanding of the issues involved and taking a definite stand in the last two sentences of the paragraph, the third giving other examples of personal restrictions in our society and raising questions about whether they are appropriate and why, and the last including a discussion of the need for pairing freedom with responsibility. The paragraph ends with a strong reiteration of the writer's point of view.

There are a few usage errors in the essay (an agreement error between "an employer" and "their employees" and a misuse of "it's"), but they do not detract from the overall strength of the essay.

Introduction to the Reading Skills Section

The Reading Skills assessment is composed of three types of questions: (1) Type I – Short Reading Passages; (2) Type II—Vocabulary in Context; and (3) Type III—Sentence Relationships. This section consists of 45 questions to be completed in 30 minutes. Note that a few "trial" questions could be scattered anywhere in this section.

Samples and Strategies

The following section will discuss and analyze each question type. Strategies are also included.

Type I: Short Reading Passages

You will be asked to analyze the ideas presented in brief passages (typically 100–150 words).

You should be able to read closely in order to

- identify important ideas
- understand direct statements
- draw inferences and conclusions
- detect underlying assumptions
- recognize word meanings in context
- respond to tone and connotation

You may be asked to select the answer choice that best summarizes a passage, explains the purpose of a passage, focuses on a specific detail, explains a word in context, compares/contrasts two aspects of a passage, explains the implications or suggestions made in a passage, identifies causal relationships, and so on.

Directions: Questions 1–5 are based on the content of short reading passages. Answer all questions following a passage on the basis of what is stated or implied in that passage.

Questions 1–2 refer to the following passage.

Because of their size and huge appetites, elephants would appear to be destructive to the environment. But in fact elephants actually use only half of the foliage they obtain from the tops of trees, leaving the rest on the ground as a food source for small ground animals. By "pruning" the plants and trees, they also stimulate new growth. In the dry season they dig holes with their forefeet, uncovering underwater springs and thus providing new watering places for themselves and other animals. Their droppings also provide food for many insects, and these insects in turn become a food source for birds. Scientists actually classify elephants as a "keystone species" because of their role in the food chain.

1. From this passage, one can infer that the term "keystone species" refers to one that

    A. is significant in maintaining an ecosystem.
    B. creates new habitats for other animals.
    C. is more valuable to mankind than other species.
    D. represents power and strength.

The best answer is **A**. The last sentence of the passage states that elephants can be classified as a keystone species because of their role in the food chain; "ecosystem" is the term that best fits this description. Choice B may seem a good answer, but the passage doesn't imply that elephants actually create new habitats for other animals, only that they uncover watering places that are used by other animals. Choice C ("more valuable to mankind") is nowhere implied in the passage, and Choice D is irrelevant. When evaluating choices, first eliminate any that are not directly relevant to the question.

2. According to this passage, which of the following is an accurate statement?

   A.   Elephants are gentler animals than assumed.

   B.   Although elephants are an endangered species, they can survive in a poor environment.

   C.   Elephants show concern for other animals by leaving foliage for them to eat.

   D.   Indirectly, elephants provide food for birds.

The best answer is **D**. See the next to the last sentence. Beware of answers that may seem correct but that go too far; for example, Choice C, on the basis of the passage, correctly states that elephants leave foliage for other animals to eat, but the words "show concern" make this answer incorrect. Nothing in the passage suggests that elephants are consciously "doing good" in the animal world. Choice A has a similar problem. The passage does say that elephants are not as destructive as assumed, but nothing implies they are "gentler." Choice B is not addressed at all in the passage.

Questions 3–5 refer to the following passage.

In the 19th century, wool was England's most valuable export, and the General Enclosure Act of 1801 standardized landlords' existing practice of fencing in open land to graze large herds of sheep. For example, in 1820 the Duchess of Sutherland dispossessed 15,000 tenants and replaced them with 131,000 sheep. One of the far-reaching effects of enclosure was that peasants, who could no longer use the open lands for their own farming, were driven into towns and cities. They became paupers with nothing to sell but their own labor, and that at whatever price the market offered. Essentially, enclosure "freed" peasants to become an army of cheap labor for the Industrial Revolution's grim new factories.

3. The probable intent of the passage is to

   A.   examine in detail the General Enclosure Act of 1801.

   B.   describe changing methods of sheep raising.

   C.   describe the effect of enclosure on the peasantry.

   D.   explain the beginnings of the Industrial Revolution.

The best answer is **C**. Starting with the second sentence, the passage deals primarily with the effect of the Enclosure Act on the peasants. The Act is not examined in detail (A). Instead, the passage presents a broad picture. The intent of the passage is to focus on the peasants, not the sheep (B), and although the writer refers to the Industrial Revolution, he/she does not "explain its beginnings" (D). When asked to determine the intent of a passage, look at the passage as a whole. Don't be misled by secondary points.

4. The writer uses the example of the Duchess of Sutherland in this passage to

   A.   dramatize the effect of enclosure on the peasants.

   B.   show the dilemma of the aristocracy.

   C.   point out that women could manage their own lands.

   D.   emphasize the success of the new method of sheep raising.

The best answer is **A**. The specific example of 15,000 peasants being displaced by 131,000 sheep dramatizes the effect of the Enclosure Act. The author of the passage uses this example to criticize the aristocracy as well, but this idea is not among the answers. Also, the rest of the passage makes it clear that the writer is not "emphasizing the success" of the new method of sheep raising (D). In answering questions about a passage, always begin by determining the writer's purpose. Choice C is completely irrelevant to the rest of the passage.

5. The word "freed" is in quotation marks because it

- **A.** is used in an informal way.
- **B.** indicates the irony of the peasants' new lives in towns and cities.
- **C.** refers to the slavery of the rural peasantry before enclosure.
- **D.** is a direct quotation from the General Enclosure Act of 1801.

The best answer is **B**. The phrase "grim new factories" is a strong clue that the author is using the term "freed" ironically. The other answers do not fit in the context of the passage. Choice C is obviously incorrect because the peasants were not slaves when they worked on the land. Nothing indicates the term "freed" appears in the Enclosure Act (D), and it is clear the author is using the term not informally (A) but ironically.

Type II: Vocabulary in Context (Replacing "Gliff" in Sentences)

You should be able to understand the meaning of a particular word or phrase in the context of a sentence.

You will be asked to consider grammatically similar words and choose the one that fits most logically into each sentence in place of a nonsense word, "gliff."

Directions: For each of questions 1–5 choose the best word or phrase to substitute for the underlined portion containing gliff, a nonsense word.

---

1. The fundamental gliff is that while oil has fueled the Arctic economy, it is the burning of such oil that has contributed to the Arctic's dangerous warming trend.

   A. cliche
   B. paradox
   C. falsity
   D. truism

The best answer is **B**. According to the statement, oil exploration in the Arctic is positive and negative at the same time—and this makes "paradox" the right choice because it means something that is seemingly contradictory and yet perhaps true. Choice A is an overused or trite phrase (and can include the concept behind the phrase); Choice C is simply an untruth; and Choice D is a completely accepted truth, one too obvious to mention. None of these is appropriate in context. In addition to having a good vocabulary, paying attention to the exact context of the word is essential in questions such as this one.

2. It was a(n) gliff stock, and she decided against buying it because she needed a steady, reliable investment.

   A. overpriced
   B. regulated
   C. volatile
   D. redundant

The best answer is **C**. The woman needs a steady, reliable investment and decided against this one because it was the opposite of steady and reliable. "Volatile," which in this context means subject to rapid or unexpected change, is therefore the best choice. A stock may be "overpriced" (A) or "regulated" (B), but neither of these is the opposite of steady and reliable. Choice D is completely irrelevant in this context. In addition to understanding the context of the missing word, a knowledge of Latin roots can be helpful.

3. The principal's method of handling the protestors was so gliff that, rather than discouraging the demonstration, it caused even more students to participate.

   A. judicious
   B. somber
   C. nebulous
   D. repressive

The best answer is **D**. In this case, "repressive" means overly severe, holding down by force. Such a method might well encourage more protestors. Choice A, which means wise or using sound judgment, or Choice B, which means gloomy or very serious, would be unlikely to do that. Choice C, meaning unclear or vague, might fit the context, but certainly not as clearly as Choice D. Remember to look for the best answer.

4. At the ceremony Randolph's leadership on the committee was praised as gliff.

    A. exemplary
    B. adequate
    C. opportune
    D. facile

The best answer is **A**. This word means commendable, worthy of imitation and praise. If Randolph's leadership were "adequate" (B), the likelihood of its inspiring praise is slight. Choice C means coming at the right time, a positive term, but not as appropriate as Choice A. And Choice D is not praiseworthy. It means shallow or too easy.

5. They looked at the painting longingly because it gliffed a time when life was simpler and sweeter.

    A. provoked
    B. evoked
    C. invoked
    D. reiterated

The best choice is **B**. It means to call forth, bring to mind, which best fits the context. Choice C is often confused with Choice B, but Choice C means (usually) to appeal to an authority, as in invoking the Constitution in a debate about free speech. Choice A is clearly wrong here and can easily be ruled out. Choice D is also inappropriate; it means to repeat or rephrase for emphasis.

Type III: Sentence Relationships (Logical Relationships)

You should be able to read two related statements and understand the relationship between them to see how

- they may contrast
- they may contradict each other
- they may show cause and effect
- one may explain the other
- one may provide a more specific example to illustrate the other
- one may explain consequence
- one may clarify something implied by the other

You will be asked to find exactly what the second sentence does in relation to the first and/or how the two sentences relate to each other.

Directions: In each of the following questions, the two underlined sentences have an implied logical relationship. Read each pair of sentences and the question that follows, and then choose the answer that identifies the relationship.

---

1. Most of the world appears to be committed to addressing global warming.

   In June of 1992 the United Nations held the Earth Summit in Rio de Janeiro to discuss stabilizing greenhouse gas concentrations in the atmosphere.

   In relation to the first sentence, what does the second sentence do?

   A. It provides support for the statement.
   B. It draws a conclusion.
   C. It introduces a different idea.
   D. It suggests an exception.

The best answer is **A**. The holding of an Earth Summit on stabilizing greenhouse gas concentrations does provide support for the statement that most of the world is committed to addressing global warming. The second sentence doesn't draw a conclusion from the first (Choice B) as much as it provides support. (In drawing conclusions, sentences will often begin with words such as "therefore".) The second sentence is directly related to the idea in the first and, therefore, C and D are poor choices.

2. Some social critics have asserted that violence in television programs contributes significantly to violence in society.

   Other commentators, however, view such programming as an "escape valve" for people's frustration and anger.

   In relation to the first sentence, what does the second sentence do?

   A. It contradicts the statement.
   B. It presents a different viewpoint.
   C. It draws a conclusion.
   D. It offers an illustration.

The best answer is **B**. A might seem the right choice, but note that the second sentence doesn't contradict the idea that some social critics hold; rather, it presents a different viewpoint. When evaluating the choices, be as precise as possible. Choices C and D can be easily ruled out.

3. <u>An alarming number of people drive around without auto insurance.</u>

<u>If one of those people hits your car and you are not sufficiently insured, you are in trouble when it comes to paying for the damage.</u>

In relation to the first sentence, what does the second sentence do?

   A. It states a consequence.
   B. It makes a comparison.
   C. It gives a reason.
   D. It draws a parallel situation.

The best answer is **A**. Sentence 2 clearly states what might happen as a result of Sentence 1. It doesn't explain why (C); neither does it make a comparison or describe a parallel situation (B, D).

4. <u>The wedding reception was more expensive than the couple had originally intended.</u>

<u>Their plans had not taken into account the number of people both sets of their parents insisted they invite.</u>

In relation to the first sentence, what does the second sentence do?

   A. It provides contrasting information.
   B. It draws the most logical inference.
   C. It supports it by giving a reason.
   D. It defines a problem.

The best choice is **C**. At first, Choice D might appear to be correct. But the second sentence doesn't define the problem stated in the first sentence. Instead, it supports the statement by giving a reason, that is, the couple had underestimated the number of people they would need to invite and therefore the reception was more expensive than they had planned. Choice A can easily be ruled out, and Choice B is inaccurate because Sentence 2 isn't "the most logical inference" from Sentence 1; the reception could have been more expensive than planned for many reasons.

5. <u>Everyone believes that the election will favor the town's most progressive elements.</u>

<u>But isn't it possible, as Harrison maintains, that a silent majority will reject the plan to sacrifice farm land for a shopping mall?</u>

In relation to the first sentence, what does the second sentence do?

   A. It identifies a cause.
   B. It questions an assumption.
   C. It explains a consequence.
   D. It presents an example.

The best answer is **B**. Sentence 1 is an assumption—that everyone believes the election will favor a particular group. Sentence 2 questions that assumption in the person of Harrison.

Sentence 2 doesn't identify the reason for the assumption in Sentence 1 (A), nor does it explain a consequence of the assumption (C). Choice D can be easily dismissed; no example is presented.

Introduction to the Composing Skills Section

The Composing Skills assessment is composed of four types of questions: (1) Type I—Construction Shift; (2) Type II—Sentence Correction; (3) Type III—Missing Sentence; and (4) Type IV—Supporting Sentence. This section consists of 45 questions to be completed in 30 minutes. Note that a few "trial" questions could be scattered anywhere in this section.

Samples and Strategies

The following section will discuss and analyze each question type. Strategies are also included.

Type I: Construction Shift (Restructuring Sentences)

You should be able to rephrase a sentence by beginning with a different construction and producing a new sentence that does not change the meaning of the original. These questions ask students to

- find a more economical or effective way of phrasing a sentence
- find a more logical way of presenting a fact or idea
- provide appropriate emphasis
- achieve sentence variety

You may be asked to spin out a sentence using an introductory phrase beginning with a gerund or an adverb, etc; or to avoid slow starts, you may be asked to consider a more appropriate noun phrase, or to consider a phrase that includes parenthetical information.

Directions: The following questions require you to rewrite sentences in your head. Each question tells you exactly how to begin your new sentence. Your new sentence should have the same meaning and contain the same information as the original sentence.

---

1. Several of the players decided to boycott the play-offs because of the committee's decision.

Rewrite, beginning with

Because of the committee's decision, . . .

The next words will be

  A. it was decided by several of the players to boycott . . .
  B. a boycott of the play-offs was decided upon by several of the players.
  C. several of the players decided to boycott . . .
  D. boycotting the play-offs was decided upon by several of the players.

The best answer is **C**. In questions where a sentence must be restructured, look for certain basic clues. For example, the active voice of the verb is generally preferred to the passive voice ("players decided" rather than "boycotting was decided by. . ."). Also, avoid the indefinite "it" when possible (Choice A).

2. An area of residential buildings was chosen by the planning commission to receive additional funds for street landscaping.

Rewrite, beginning with

The planning commission . . .

The next words will be

A. was responsible for choosing . . .
B. in choosing where to apply additional funds chose . . .
C. had been chosen to receive additional funds . . .
D. chose an area of residential buildings to receive . . .

The best answer is **D**. Again, as in sample 1, choose the active voice. Also, avoid answers that lack clarity; for example, Choice C is structured so that the planning commission is the object of the choice rather than the chooser.

Other things to watch for in restructuring sentences: Does the answer change the meaning of the original sentence (as choices A and C do in this case)? Is a choice too wordy (as Choice B is)?

3. The actress forgot her lines in the middle of the play, which caused the audience to break into nervous laughter.

Rewrite, beginning with

The audience broke into nervous laughter . . .

The next words will be

A. caused by the actress, who forgot her lines.
B. when the actress forgot her lines.
C. in the middle of the play caused by the actress who forgot.
D. causing the actress to forget her lines.

The best answer is **B**. Choice B is the most direct version of the sentence. Both choices A and C are wordy, and choice D changes the meaning of the original sentence.

4. As a surprise for his grandparents, Jonathan had booked passage on a luxury cruise ship headed for Tahiti.

Rewrite, beginning with

Jonathan had booked passage . . .

A. on a luxury cruise ship, as a surprise for his grandparents, headed for Tahiti.
B. on a luxury cruise ship headed for Tahiti, as a surprise for his grandparents.
C. as a surprise for his grandparents headed for Tahiti on a luxury cruise ship.
D. in order to surprise his grandparents on a luxury cruise ship headed for Tahiti.

The best answer is **B**. Choice B keeps related elements of the sentence together: "on a luxury cruise ship headed for Tahiti". Choice A awkwardly divides the related elements: "luxury cruise ship, as a surprise for his grandparents, headed for Tahiti". Choices C and D both suggest that the grandparents received the surprise while they were already on the cruise. Also, Choice D includes an unnecessary phrase ("in order to"). Avoid phrases that lengthen a sentence without adding meaning.

5. To ski in the Alps and swim in the Adriatic were dreams that Joanna cherished all her life.

Rewrite, beginning with

All her life . . .

- **A.** Joanna cherished dreams of skiing in the Alps and swimming in the Adriatic.
- **B.** Joanna's cherished dreams were of skiing in the Alps and to swim in the Adriatic.
- **C.** Joanna cherished dreams, which were of skiing in the Alps and of swimming in the Adriatic.
- **D.** to ski in the Alps and swimming in the Adriatic were the dreams that Joanna cherished.

The best answer is **A**. Both choices B and D are examples of faulty parallelism: "skiing and swimming" are parallel grammatically; while "of skiing and to swim" and "to ski and swimming" are not. Choice C is wordy.

Type II: Sentence Correction (Selecting the Best Version of a Sentence)

You should be able to find the best way of correcting a sentence in order to resolve problems of

- clarity
- sentence predication
- parallel structure
- subordination and coordination
- modification
- sentence boundaries

You are asked to select the best way to phrase an underlined portion of a sentence. This question type tests the your understanding of syntax, usage, and idiom rather than specific knowledge of grammatical rules.

Directions: In each of the following questions, select the best version of the underlined part of the sentence. Choice A is the same as the underlined portion of the original sentence. If you think the original sentence is best, choose A.

---

1. Jonas Salk, who developed the first successful polio vaccine, and he used the newly developed tissue culture method of working with the virus.

   A. and he used
   B. using
   C. , used
   D. , which used

The best answer is **C**. The original sentence (A) is a fragment because the first clause has no predicate (main verb). Choices B and D are also fragments. In questions like these, first read all the choices carefully to make sure that one of them is grammatically complete, that is, has a subject and predicate and expresses a complete thought. Don't be misled by clauses that can't stand alone or by forms of the verb that cannot act alone as a predicate (for example, "using" in Choice B).

2. To economize during cold weather, weather stripping that is backed with adhesive and then applied around doors and windows.

   A. weather stripping that is backed with adhesive and then applied around doors and windows.
   B. you can apply weather stripping with adhesive backing around doors and windows.
   C. around doors and windows and with adhesive backing weather stripping can be applied.
   D. applying weather stripping using adhesive backing around doors and windows.

The best answer is **B**. Notice the subject ("you") and the predicate ("can apply"). Once again, choices A and D are fragments. Choice C is not a fragment, but it is awkwardly constructed. And all choices other than B leave out the person who is economizing, you. In questions like these, after determining which choices are complete sentences, select the one that is least awkward or wordy.

3. After World War II, colleges and universities were swamped with applications, and they expected a different kind of education.

   A. and they expected
   B. and the applicants expected
   C. who expected
   D. which were expectant of

The best answer is **B**. In the original sentence (Choice A), and in choices C and D, it appears that the "applications" or the "colleges" are doing the expecting. The problem here is that the pronouns ("they," "who," and "which") have no correct antecedent (the word for which a pronoun stands—in this case "applicants").

---

4. The word "thesaurus", which derives from a Latin word meaning "treasure," so that literally a thesaurus is a storehouse or treasury of words.

    A. , which derives from
    B. , derived from
    C. , deriving from
    D. is derived from

The best answer is **D**. The original sentence and choices B and C are fragments. Although Choice D is in the passive voice, it is the only choice that makes the sentence complete. Notice that the comma must be eliminated.

---

5. During the storm dozens of families were evacuated from low-lying areas, an action which required careful coordination of resources by the authorities.

    A. an action that required careful coordination
    B. it required careful coordination
    C. careful coordination of resources by the authorities was required for this action
    D. for which was required careful coordination

The best answer is **A**. In this case, the original version of the sentence, is the best answer. Choices B and C are run-on sentences (two sentences run together without proper punctuation or without a coordinating conjunction such as "and"). Run-on sentences are also called comma splices. Choice D is wordy and awkward.

Type III: Missing Sentence (Choosing the Missing Sentence)

You should be able to select an appropriate sentence that most logically

- begins a paragraph
- fits in the middle of a paragraph
- ends a paragraph

You may be asked to find the most appropriate topic sentence (one that most successfully generalizes what follows); to find the most appropriate middle sentence (adds specifics or carries the paragraph forward in some way); or to find the sentence that logically concludes the paragraph.

Directions: Each of the following questions presents a passage with a missing sentence indicated by a series of dashes. Read each passage and the four sentences that follow it. Then choose the sentence that can best be inserted in place of the dashes.

---

1. Henry Petroski, a professor of civil engineering, believes that many less-than-perfect designs aren't caused by human error but rather by the impossibility of making design choices that satisfy all constraints. A thick toothbrush would be easy to manipulate, for example, but would not fit in traditional bathroom racks. - - - - - - -. According to Petroski, all designs involve such trade-offs.

   A. Therefore, the designer must compromise the design by considering compatibility with the world as it currently exists.
   B. The design of a toothbrush is a trivial concern that doesn't require extensive engineering expertise.
   C. However, many people use electric or battery-powered toothbrushes.
   D. It is fascinating to study all the factors involved in designing simple items, and it gives one an appreciation for the talents of designers.

The best answer is **A**. Directly related to the first sentence and leading to the last sentence, it clarifies Petroski's point. In the passage, the toothbrush is a specific example; choices B and C, while relevant to toothbrushes, are not relevant to the main idea of the passage. Choice D introduces a different point altogether—appreciation for designers' talents. With this type of question, don't choose answers that relate to trivial or extraneous matters or lead in a different direction.

---

2. - - - - - - -. Thomas Bullfinch compiled the three volumes of his classical work on mythology to point out how many important authors were inspired by myths and legends. Among the most famous were Shakespeare, Milton, Dante, and Longfellow. Modern authors have continued the tradition, sometimes basing entire works on classical myths, usually updated to appeal to a contemporary audience.

   A. Myths and legends have always intrigued people, including young children, who love the heroic tales.
   B. It is well known that Sigmund Freud based his psychoanalytical thinking on the myth of Oedipus.
   C. Studying classical mythology can be fun as well as illuminating.
   D. Classical myths and legends are an integral part of Western literature.

The best answer is **D**. It is an appropriate topic sentence for the passage, which deals specifically with the influence of myths on literature. Choice C, in addition to being an uninteresting sentence, isn't precisely on the topic. Choices A and B may both be true, but they do not introduce the subject of the passage.

3. Learning to appreciate small towns can be a challenge. When I was a child, my parents followed their dream of giving up the hectic pace of New York to run a small farm in a remote (at least to me) town in Iowa. - - - - - - -. But when I was given a calf to raise, all my complaints about our new life disappeared.

   A. Family farms are a risky business, with large agricultural corporations dominating the scene.
   B. At first, rural charms left me cold.
   C. My old friends from the apartment building in New York promised to visit me.
   D. My mother's family was from Iowa, and she had never been happy in the "big city".

The best answer is **B**. Both the first and last sentences provide a clue. In the first, the writer refers to the challenge of living in a small town and in the last mentions his/her complaints. The word "But" in the last sentence is also a clue. The passage as a whole deals with the writer's adjustment to rural life and has nothing to do with the risks of farming (A) or his/her mother's background (D).

4. The first humans gathered plants and hunted animals much like the other herbivorous and carnivorous animals around them. Although they were able to devise tools and weapons and create a social organization that made hunting and food gathering easier, at this point they didn't have much impact on the environment. - - - - - - -.

   A. Humans were more intelligent than other animals, in spite of the fact that they were smaller and physically weaker.
   B. The earliest tools were primitive and awkward to use, but thanks to their intelligence, humans developed industrial processes that led to improvements in tool-making.
   C. Cro-magnon man appeared in Europe towards the end of the Pleistocene ice age.
   D. The first great change occurred when humans, rather than hunting and gathering, began to bring animals and plants together in one location, clearing more and more land of its natural vegetation.

The best answer is **D**. The passage leads to a statement about the effect of humans on the environment. The words "first great change" in this sentence indicate its relationship to the previous two. Choice B, while it may seem relevant, is focused on tool-making, not on the environment, whereas both choices A and C are off the subject.

5. According to a popular belief, Columbus had to convince King Ferdinand and Queen Isabella that the world was round, not flat, so that they would underwrite his voyage to the New World. The truth is, however, that the ancient Greeks had already discovered that the earth was a sphere. - - - - - - -. What Columbus did have to do was offer the king and queen an estimate of the earth's circumference.

   A. In addition to their achievements in mathematics and philosophy, the Greeks were knowledgeable about astronomy and geography.
   B. The question of the earth's position in the solar system was much more problematical and much less likely to be solved.
   C. By Columbus's time most educated people also believed the earth was round.
   D. It took Columbus eight years to convince King Ferdinand and Queen Isabella to finance his trip.

The best answer is **C**. It connects smoothly to the sentence that precedes it (note the use of the word "also") and supports the idea that the "popular belief" in the first sentence is inaccurate. Choices A and B are irrelevant to the subject of Columbus. Choice D is more relevant, but the length of time it took Columbus to convince the king and queen is not tied to the first two sentences.

Type IV: Supporting Sentence (Choosing a Sentence That Provides Support)

You should be able to read a sentence and decide which of four subsequent sentences will give appropriate logical support by

- adding relevant detail
- stating a probable cause or explanation
- providing a supporting example

You will be asked to discriminate among sentences that might all seem related to the original sentence, but only one of which provides logical support for the original.

Directions: Each of the following questions presents a topic and four sentences. Select the sentence that provides the best support for the topic presented.

---

1. The movie industry continues to change as film makers explore new technology.

    A. Generally, "blockbuster" action movies are more popular with men than with women.
    B. The movie rating system has proved to be valuable to parents who want to protect their children from films with adult content.
    C. Movie attendance is affected dramatically when a studio actively promotes a particular film.
    D. Special effects have become more and more dramatic and inventive in recent years.

The best answer is **D**. The topic sentence specifies changes due to "new technology." Of the possible answers, choice D is the only one that directly relates to technology as it is applied by film makers. Film promotion (C) may be changed by technological advances, but the topic sentence specifies the role of film makers, not film promoters. An important thing to remember in answering this type of question: While all of the choices might vaguely relate to the general subject, choose the one that very specifically supports the topic.

2. In the United States, dependence on fossil fuels has become a major problem both politically and environmentally.

    A. In some areas, such as the Arctic, oil exploration threatens to destroy the habitats of wild animals..
    B. Many people prefer riding mass transit to driving because it offers the chance for a little nap before the workday begins.
    C. Hybrid cars get significantly higher mileage than traditional cars.
    D. Our grandparents talk nostalgically of a time when gasoline was cheap and gas station attendants offered to check the air in the tires and clean the windshield.

The best answer is **A**. The topic sentence deals with the "problem both politically and environmentally" of dependence on fossil fuels. Choice A supports this statement by pointing out the dangers to "habitats of wild animals" in the Arctic— clearly an environmental issue. Choice C mentions a possible way to decrease fossil fuel dependency but is not evidence for the statement in the topic sentence. Both choices B and D are irrelevant.

3. The author's position is that history followed different courses for different populations in the world not because of biological differences but because of various conditions in the environments of each population.

    A. Most Polynesian islands are surrounded by shallow water and reefs.
    B. Societies are different on each of the Polynesian islands as a result of variables such as climate, geological type, marine resources, area, and degree of isolation.
    C. The most productive Polynesian agriculture was the cultivation of taro fields, although taro was not the only crop the Polynesians produced.
    D. Ancestral Polynesians brought with them three domesticated animals (the pig, chicken, and dog) and domesticated no further animals within Polynesia.

The best answer is **B**. What is the main idea in the first sentence? Different environmental conditions, not different biological factors, account for differences in the history of populations. Choice B specifically cites environmental factors (climate, geological type, etc.) as a cause of the variations among societies on the different Polynesian islands and is therefore supporting the topic sentence. Choices A, C, and D, make no reference to differences among populations or the cause of those differences.

---

4. After I moved out of my parents' home into my own apartment, I learned about responsibility the hard way.

   A. Most of the furniture I acquired came from a variety of thrift shops and secondhand stores, but it was comfortable and satisfied my needs.

   B. The couple who lived down the hall from me spent most of their time arguing at the top of their lungs, and I considered offering to be their marriage counselor.

   C. When I didn't pay my rent on time, my landlord charged me an outrageously high "late fee" and told me if it happened again, I might be out on my ear.

   D. Frozen dinners and fast-food every night of the week didn't begin to measure up to my mother's gourmet meals.

The best answer is **C**. This sentence most clearly supports the idea of "learning about responsibility the hard way." Choice A is a positive statement, and while choices B and D are negative points about moving into his/her own apartment, neither is related to learning about responsibility.

---

5. Whether you use a digital camera or an "old-fashioned" one, try to avoid trite photographs of well-known landmarks and spectacular views.

   A. Digital cameras are available at different prices, depending on whether you are satisfied with being an amateur or aspire to being a professional.

   B. Consider taking photos under unusual conditions of weather and lighting, for example.

   C. If you are using an old camera, be sure to choose the speed of your film carefully.

   D. Editing digital photos can be both fun and challenging for beginners.

The correct answer is **B**. Notice that the topic sentence is about avoiding trite photographs, not about the type of camera to use. Taking photos under "unusual conditions" would help to avoid triteness. Choices A, C, and D are specifically related to the type of camera, not to the quality of the photos.

PART V

SIMULATED EPT PRACTICE TEST

The EPT has three sections—one essay, a multiple-choice reading skills section (45 questions), and a multiple-choice composing skills section (45 questions). There are "trial" questions that can be scattered throughout each multiple-choice section. These are being tested for future exams. This simulated practice exam is followed by complete explanations.

Remember, the time limits are:

- essay—45 minutes
- multiple-choice reading skills section—30 minutes
- multiple-choice composing skills section—30 minutes

The problems in this simulated practice exam are designed to be similar in structure, style, variety, and difficulty level to the problems on the actual exam. The actual EPT is copyrighted and may not be duplicated. These questions are not taken from the actual test.

Answer Sheets for Practice Test

(Remove This Sheet and Use It to Mark Your Answers)

Reading Skills

Part A

1 Ⓐ Ⓑ Ⓒ Ⓓ
2 Ⓐ Ⓑ Ⓒ Ⓓ
3 Ⓐ Ⓑ Ⓒ Ⓓ
4 Ⓐ Ⓑ Ⓒ Ⓓ
5 Ⓐ Ⓑ Ⓒ Ⓓ
6 Ⓐ Ⓑ Ⓒ Ⓓ
7 Ⓐ Ⓑ Ⓒ Ⓓ
8 Ⓐ Ⓑ Ⓒ Ⓓ
9 Ⓐ Ⓑ Ⓒ Ⓓ
10 Ⓐ Ⓑ Ⓒ Ⓓ
11 Ⓐ Ⓑ Ⓒ Ⓓ
12 Ⓐ Ⓑ Ⓒ Ⓓ
13 Ⓐ Ⓑ Ⓒ Ⓓ
14 Ⓐ Ⓑ Ⓒ Ⓓ
15 Ⓐ Ⓑ Ⓒ Ⓓ

Part B

16 Ⓐ Ⓑ Ⓒ Ⓓ
17 Ⓐ Ⓑ Ⓒ Ⓓ
18 Ⓐ Ⓑ Ⓒ Ⓓ
19 Ⓐ Ⓑ Ⓒ Ⓓ
20 Ⓐ Ⓑ Ⓒ Ⓓ
21 Ⓐ Ⓑ Ⓒ Ⓓ
22 Ⓐ Ⓑ Ⓒ Ⓓ
23 Ⓐ Ⓑ Ⓒ Ⓓ
24 Ⓐ Ⓑ Ⓒ Ⓓ
25 Ⓐ Ⓑ Ⓒ Ⓓ
26 Ⓐ Ⓑ Ⓒ Ⓓ
27 Ⓐ Ⓑ Ⓒ Ⓓ
28 Ⓐ Ⓑ Ⓒ Ⓓ
29 Ⓐ Ⓑ Ⓒ Ⓓ
30 Ⓐ Ⓑ Ⓒ Ⓓ

Part C

31 Ⓐ Ⓑ Ⓒ Ⓓ
32 Ⓐ Ⓑ Ⓒ Ⓓ
33 Ⓐ Ⓑ Ⓒ Ⓓ
34 Ⓐ Ⓑ Ⓒ Ⓓ
35 Ⓐ Ⓑ Ⓒ Ⓓ
36 Ⓐ Ⓑ Ⓒ Ⓓ
37 Ⓐ Ⓑ Ⓒ Ⓓ
38 Ⓐ Ⓑ Ⓒ Ⓓ
39 Ⓐ Ⓑ Ⓒ Ⓓ
40 Ⓐ Ⓑ Ⓒ Ⓓ
41 Ⓐ Ⓑ Ⓒ Ⓓ
42 Ⓐ Ⓑ Ⓒ Ⓓ
43 Ⓐ Ⓑ Ⓒ Ⓓ
44 Ⓐ Ⓑ Ⓒ Ⓓ
45 Ⓐ Ⓑ Ⓒ Ⓓ

CUT HERE

Composing Skills

Part A

1 Ⓐ Ⓑ Ⓒ Ⓓ
2 Ⓐ Ⓑ Ⓒ Ⓓ
3 Ⓐ Ⓑ Ⓒ Ⓓ
4 Ⓐ Ⓑ Ⓒ Ⓓ
5 Ⓐ Ⓑ Ⓒ Ⓓ
6 Ⓐ Ⓑ Ⓒ Ⓓ
7 Ⓐ Ⓑ Ⓒ Ⓓ
8 Ⓐ Ⓑ Ⓒ Ⓓ
9 Ⓐ Ⓑ Ⓒ Ⓓ
10 Ⓐ Ⓑ Ⓒ Ⓓ
11 Ⓐ Ⓑ Ⓒ Ⓓ
12 Ⓐ Ⓑ Ⓒ Ⓓ

Part B

13 Ⓐ Ⓑ Ⓒ Ⓓ
14 Ⓐ Ⓑ Ⓒ Ⓓ
15 Ⓐ Ⓑ Ⓒ Ⓓ
16 Ⓐ Ⓑ Ⓒ Ⓓ
17 Ⓐ Ⓑ Ⓒ Ⓓ
18 Ⓐ Ⓑ Ⓒ Ⓓ
19 Ⓐ Ⓑ Ⓒ Ⓓ
20 Ⓐ Ⓑ Ⓒ Ⓓ
21 Ⓐ Ⓑ Ⓒ Ⓓ
22 Ⓐ Ⓑ Ⓒ Ⓓ
23 Ⓐ Ⓑ Ⓒ Ⓓ
24 Ⓐ Ⓑ Ⓒ Ⓓ
25 Ⓐ Ⓑ Ⓒ Ⓓ

Part C

26 Ⓐ Ⓑ Ⓒ Ⓓ
27 Ⓐ Ⓑ Ⓒ Ⓓ
28 Ⓐ Ⓑ Ⓒ Ⓓ
29 Ⓐ Ⓑ Ⓒ Ⓓ
30 Ⓐ Ⓑ Ⓒ Ⓓ
31 Ⓐ Ⓑ Ⓒ Ⓓ
32 Ⓐ Ⓑ Ⓒ Ⓓ
33 Ⓐ Ⓑ Ⓒ Ⓓ
34 Ⓐ Ⓑ Ⓒ Ⓓ
35 Ⓐ Ⓑ Ⓒ Ⓓ
36 Ⓐ Ⓑ Ⓒ Ⓓ

Part D

37 Ⓐ Ⓑ Ⓒ Ⓓ
38 Ⓐ Ⓑ Ⓒ Ⓓ
39 Ⓐ Ⓑ Ⓒ Ⓓ
40 Ⓐ Ⓑ Ⓒ Ⓓ
41 Ⓐ Ⓑ Ⓒ Ⓓ
42 Ⓐ Ⓑ Ⓒ Ⓓ
43 Ⓐ Ⓑ Ⓒ Ⓓ
44 Ⓐ Ⓑ Ⓒ Ⓓ
45 Ⓐ Ⓑ Ⓒ Ⓓ

CUT HERE

Practice Test

Directions: You will have 45 minutes to plan and write an essay on the topic assigned below. Before you begin writing, read the passage carefully and plan what you will say. Your essay should be as well organized and as carefully written as you can make it.

"This has been hailed as the 'information age,' as though we live at the best of times in a utopia where having "information" will make us all suddenly happy, healthy, wealthy, and wise. But in many ways, we might well be better off without this information overload. From morning till night we are bombarded with supposed facts, opinions, and just plain noise to the extent that there is rarely time to actually think."

—Colin Magnus

Explain Magnus's argument and discuss the extent to which you agree or disagree with his analysis. Support your position, providing reasons and examples from your own experience, observations, or reading.

Reading Skills

30 Minutes

45 Questions

Part A

Directions: Questions 1–15 are based on the content of short reading passages. Answer all questions following a passage on the basis of what is stated or implied in that passage.

Questions 1–4 are based on the following passage.

Peter Roget put together his thesaurus in 1852, and some high school teachers think he might have created a monster. Yes, Roget's Thesaurus can be a helpful dictionary of synonyms. But it can also lead students into egregious errors when they use it. A naive writer might well choose a synonym that is pretentious or one that is quite wrong in context. Roget's creation might be a monster in another way, too. He organized the words elaborately, creating fifteen classes (such as "Feelings" and "Behaviour and the Will"), and many sections (like "revulsion" or "newness") within the classes. To find synonyms for a word, the user must first find the word in an alphabetical index and then turn to the proper class and section. A modern A-Z thesaurus is much easier and quicker to use. Still, a student might choose an inappropriate word—"verbose" to describe a talkative teenager, for example.

1. From the passage one can infer that the word "egregious" means

   A. amusing and lively.
   B. unnecessarily provocative.
   C. conspicuously bad.
   D. argumentative and confrontational.

2. The author of the passages implies that Roget's Thesaurus is

   A. inconveniently organized.
   B. useless.
   C. overly praised.
   D. inadequately researched.

3. The purpose of the last sentence of the passage is to

   A. give an example of the limitations of any thesaurus.
   B. criticize Roget for his method in preparing his thesaurus.
   C. emphasize the importance of dictionaries.
   D. change the tone of the passage.

4. Which of the following sentences is figurative rather than literal?

   A. A naive writer might well choose a synonym . . . .
   B. . . . some high school teachers think he might have created a monster.
   C. . . . the user must find the word in an alphabetical index . . . .
   D. He organized the words elaborately, creating fifteen classes . . . .

Questions 5–8 are based on the following passage.

For many years, Niagara Falls—a traditional honeymoon spot—was the home of a shriveled mummy with crossed arms that could be the remains of long-lost Egyptian ruler. The story of how he ended up on a dusty museum shelf is murky, involving looting, illegal purchase, and neglect. Dr. James Douglas originally acquired a mummy collection for the Niagara Falls Museum. Fascinated by Egyptian culture, Douglas even displayed mummies on his front porch. The museum collection was a hit, attracting people like Abraham Lincoln, Ulysses S. Grant, and P.T. Barnum. Suspicions that the crossed-armed mummy might be a noble arose decades ago, but in the 1960s, the suggestions were declared unfounded. It wasn't until 1998 when the Niagara museum closed down and the mummies went to Emory University that an expert, through a background check including CT scans and X-ray images, declared that the mummy was a king. One candidate stood out: Rameses I, founder of the 19th dynasty of Egypt's illustrious new kingdom. Where is the mummy today? It has been brought home to rest in the Cairo Museum, where the mummies of Rameses' family are housed.

5. The author's use of the phrase "a traditional honeymoon spot" in the first sentence is most likely to

   A. help the reader locate the site of the museum.
   B. show that Niagara Falls has many attractions.
   C. emphasize that one wouldn't expect to find mummies in Niagara Falls.
   D. poke fun at the people who honeymoon in Niagara Falls.

6. In the passage the author's primary purpose is to

   A. tell a historical anecdote.
   B. show the dangers of looting ancient tombs.
   C. illustrate the popularity of Egyptian culture.
   D. show proof that the mummy is Rameses I.

7. The author implies in the passage that

   A. Dr. James Douglas looted an Egyptian tomb.
   B. mummies were a popular attraction in the United States.
   C. the mummy may not be Rameses I.
   D. Cairo fought vigorously for the return of the mummy.

8. In the context of the passage, "murky" means

   A. surprisingly lucky.
   B. reprehensible.
   C. darkly obscure.
   D. not researched.

GO ON TO THE NEXT PAGE

Questions 9–12 are based on the following passage.

The Peruvian site of Machu Picchu is 7,720 feet above sea level, and not easy to get to. For the last 1,640 vertical feet, a visitor must walk over the course of several days up steps, through tunnels, and across bridges. This city in the sky, with terraces connected by footpaths and ancient Incan structures, is a place where the traveler can get a glimpse of pre-Columbian South America. In 1911 Hiram Bingham of Yale University "rediscovered" it. He was in search of the "lost city of the Incas," and thought he had found it. But today experts say Machu Picchu is not the fabled "lost city." Instead, it was probably a retreat for the Incan emperor. Since its discovery, Machu Picchu's accessibility has been a mixed blessing. In 1999, preservationists were outraged at the plan to build a cable car lift for tourists, and in September of 2000 a huge sundial known as the "Hitching Post of the Sun" was damaged during filming of a beer commercial. If the emperor were to return, how would he react to the popularity of his retreat?

9. The tone of the passage can best be described as

   A. reverent.
   B. factual.
   C. ironic.
   D. sentimental.

10. The phrase "mixed blessing" refers to the fact that

   A. tourism has benefitted the rich but not the poor in Machu Picchu.
   B. Machu Picchu is not the "lost city" but only an Incan fortress.
   C. the discovery of Machu Picchu has had both positive and negative results.
   D. the trip to Machu Picchu is both difficult and rewarding.

11. The last sentence of the passage

   A. asks a rhetorical question.
   B. introduces an argument.
   C. underlines the main idea of the passage.
   D. questions the passage's point of view.

12. The phrase "fabled lost city of the Incas" implies that

   A. most people believe in the "lost city."
   B. the Incas cleverly hid some of their cities.
   C. the city may or may not exist.
   D. no one will ever find the real "lost city."

Questions 13–15 are based on the following passage.

Too many patents are granted in the United States. Ninety-five percent of patent applications are approved, compared to 65 percent in Europe and Japan. In part, understaffing in the United States patent office is the culprit. Because examiners have such a heavy load of applications to review, they don't have enough time to thoroughly research an idea's originality. They are inclined to make decisions favorable to the applicant. According to some people, granting many patents is a good thing because it encourages innovation. If inventors know they can receive the protection that a patent grants, they will be encouraged to create. However, studies suggest that this isn't the case. For example, countries that have strengthened their patent protection have not seen an increase in innovation.

13. The author's purpose in this passage is to

  A. describe the patent system in the United States.
  B. compare the patent system in the United States with systems in other countries.
  C. explain the effect of granting too many patents.
  D. suggest that patents are awarded too easily in the United States.

14. Some people believe that the protection provided by a patent will encourage innovation because

  A. it shows that the government is a strong supporter of innovation.
  B. people will take new inventions more seriously.
  C. it promises greater financial gain for the inventor.
  D. it weeds out poor ideas.

15. The author of the passage does NOT

  A. explain why too many patents are a bad idea.
  B. make comparisons.
  C. suggest a reason that so many patents are granted.
  D. reveal a point of view.

GO ON TO THE NEXT PAGE

Part B

Directions: For each of the following questions choose the best word or phrase to substitute for the underlined portion containing gliff, a nonsense word.

16. Her gliff smile convinced him she was as innocent and sweet as she seemed.

    A. absent-minded
    B. flirtatious
    C. winsome
    D. triumphant

17. Harriet's gliff remarks bored everyone to tears.

    A. insipid
    B. angry
    C. spontaneous
    D. vicious

18. She had been gliff for so long that even the walk to the store wore her out.

    A. dreaming
    B. languid
    C. sedentary
    D. cautious

19. The background of the painting was gliff, more like a wild dream than a peaceful landscape.

    A. ambivalent
    B. putrid
    C. inconsequential
    D. surrealistic

20. Although she clung gliff to her belief in her brother's innocence, Rosalind listened to all the charges against him.

    A. tenaciously
    B. subtly
    C. logically
    D. spiritually

21. Driving back to the farm, I already missed the gliff atmosphere of the city.

    A. literate
    B. congested
    C. gentrified
    D. cosmopolitan

22. For many years the faculty of the small college was a gliff group, but the issue of dropping the humanities course caused a serious rift.

- A. personable
- B. congenial
- C. polarized
- D. solemn

23. Nothing the actor said would make the magazine gliff its story about his recklessness.

- A. reposition
- B. negate
- C. retract
- D. decrease

24. Because the manager didn't want to gliff progress on the building, he agreed to the contractor's changes.

- A. impede
- B. mock
- C. propel
- D. shatter

25. The regulations concerning contamination were gliff, and the factory owner wasn't sure his operation could comply with them.

- A. potent
- B. miserly
- C. stringent
- D. fruitless

26. The book included a gliff account of the hero's death, and Joanne found herself close to tears.

- A. repulsive
- B. poignant
- C. graceful
- D. realistic

27. David's asking her father's permission to marry her seemed an gliff custom to Pamela, who had lived on her own for 10 years.

- A. opportune
- B. insane
- C. unwieldy
- D. archaic

GO ON TO THE NEXT PAGE

28. After a series of gliffs that tested every aspect of his character and strength, the handsome stranger won the hand of the princess.

    A. travails
    B. days
    C. riddles
    D. touchstones

29. The speech should gliff the cocktail hour and the dinner.

    A. proceed
    B. overtake
    C. precede
    D. preclude

30. His friends admired Carlos's gliff in stating that he felt his experiment was flawed.

    A. sarcasm
    B. humility
    C. logic
    D. candor

Part C

Directions: In each of the following questions, the two underlined sentences have an implied logical relationship. Read each pair of sentences and the question that follows, and then choose the answer that identifies the relationship.

31. The gap in pay between people with skills and people without them seems to be widening.

    The pay difference between women of varied mathematical skills had grown from $.93 an hour in 1978 to $1.71 and hour in 1986.

    In relation to the first sentence, what does the second sentence do?

    A. It provides an example.
    B. It draws a conclusion.
    C. It introduces a different idea.
    D. It suggests an exception.

32. Polls indicate that many Americans believe the Internet should be regulated by the government.

    But is this really a good idea?

    In relation to the first sentence, what does the second sentence do?

    A. It makes a comparison.
    B. It suggests an exception.
    C. It introduces a different point of view.
    D. It refutes the statement.

33. In his determination to avenge his father, Hamlet cruelly disdained Ophelia.

    Broken-hearted, she went mad and drowned herself.

    In relation to the first sentence, what does the second sentence do?

    A. It offers an illustration.
    B. It supports the statement.
    C. It defines a problem.
    D. It states an effect.

34. The United States is losing its old-growth forests at an alarming rate.

    Wood consumption has increased 30 percent since 1930.

    In relation to the first sentence, what does the second sentence do?

    A. It gives an example.
    B. It presents a reason.
    C. It questions an assumption.
    D. It provides a contrast.

GO ON TO THE NEXT PAGE

35. The first half of the play was witty and clever, and the audience loved every minute.

The second half fell flat, and the theater was silent as a tomb.

In relation to the first sentence, what does the second sentence do?

   A. It presents a contrast.
   B. It offers an illustration.
   C. It refutes an idea.
   D. It explains a consequence.

36. When I was a child, I had difficulty making friends.

Just as I would be getting to know someone, my father would announce we were moving.

In relation to the first sentence, what does the second sentence do?

   A. It draws a parallel.
   B. It makes a comparison.
   C. It gives supporting evidence.
   D. It suggests a cause.

37. The Supreme Court's fundamental purpose is to commit the United States to the rule of law rather than to the rule of individual men.

During the Civil War, Abraham Lincoln suspended the *writ of habeas corpus,* and the Court invalidated the suspension.

In relation to the first sentence, what does the second sentence do?

   A. It gives a reason.
   B. It suggests a cause.
   C. It supports the statement.
   D. It makes a comparison.

38. Some science fiction novels present a darkly pessimistic view of the future.

They are filled with gloomy predictions of where technology will ultimately lead mankind.

In relation to the first sentence, what does the second sentence do?

   A. It provides emphasis.
   B. It makes an exception.
   C. It gives supporting evidence.
   D. It draws a conclusion.

39. Ten years ago my family lived in a tiny apartment in the worst part of town.

Today, we own our own spacious home in a pleasant suburban community.

In relation to the first sentence, what does the second sentence do?

A. It draws a conclusion.
B. It makes a comparison.
C. It states a consequence.
D. It gives supporting evidence.

40. The most successful schools in America are in affluent communities.

The kids at Rockford, a small country high school, would dispute that generalization.

In relation to the first sentence, what does the second sentence do?

A. It questions an assumption.
B. It makes a comparison.
C. It provides emphasis.
D. It introduces a new subject.

41. The new recreation center offers a wide variety of activities at reasonable costs.

Community members can take lessons in such things as tap dancing, tai chi, swimming, making pottery, and so on, and all at fees half as much as private lessons would cost.

In relation to the first sentence, what does the second sentence do?

A. It states a consequence.
B. It gives examples.
C. It makes a comparison.
D. It suggests a cause.

42. Four apartment houses were destroyed in the explosion.

Families wandered aimlessly in the streets, not knowing where to go or whom to turn to for help.

In relation to the first sentence, what does the second sentence do?

A. It gives an example.
B. It suggests a cause.
C. It states a consequence.
D. It provides emphasis.

GO ON TO THE NEXT PAGE

43. Everyone at the meeting showed enthusiastic support for the plan to expand the skateboard park.

But old Mr. Martin, who came in late and stood at the back of the room, shook his head emphatically and then stormed out.

In relation to the first sentence, what does the second sentence do?

A. It provides emphasis.
B. It gives an example.
C. It suggests a consequence.
D. It notes an exception.

44. Despite significant changes to the landscape in recent years, the park still teems with diverse life.

More than a thousand species of plants thrive, and wildlife residents include the badger, coyote, mountain lion, and sixteen species of bats.

In relation to the first sentence, what does the second sentence do?

A. It suggests a cause.
B. It gives supporting evidence.
C. It introduces a different point of view.
D. It refutes an assumption.

45. Some people believe that the city was founded in the spirit of community and a shared mission, with everyone working together to produce splendid buildings.

It is more likely that it was a city run by the rich and powerful who forced less fortunate men into constructing huge palaces.

In relation to the first sentence, what does the second sentence do?

A. It questions an assumption.
B. It makes a comparison.
C. It provides an example
D. It adds emphasis.

IF YOU FINISH BEFORE TIME IS CALLED, CHECK YOUR WORK ON THIS SECTION ONLY. DO NOT WORK ON ANY OTHER SECTION IN THE TEST.

Composing Skills

30 Minutes

45 Questions

Part A

Directions: The following questions require you to rewrite sentences in your head. Each question tells you exactly how to begin your new sentence. Your new sentence should have the same meaning and contain the same information as the original sentence.

1. The hikers gathered at the foot of the mountain and listened to the ranger's warnings.

   Rewrite, beginning with

   Having gathered at the foot of the mountain, ...

   The next words will be

   A. the ranger's warnings
   B. the hikers
   C. warnings from the ranger
   D. they

2. An early arrival in Philadelphia was confidently predicted by the pilot because he counted on strong tail winds.

   Rewrite, beginning with

   The pilot confidently predicted . . . .

   The next words will be

   A. strong tail winds
   B. it would be
   C. an early arrival
   D. they could count on

3. Some committee members, wanting to achieve agreement by the end of the meeting, reluctantly decided to compromise on the issue.

   Rewrite, beginning with

   Because they wanted to achieve agreement by the end of the meeting, ...

   The next words will be

   A. a reluctant decision
   B. a compromise on the issue
   C. it was decided by
   D. some committee members decided

4. A group of students from Argentina was chosen by the sponsor of the event to lead the delegation that would attend the final ceremony.

   Rewrite, beginning with

   To lead the delegation that would attend the final ceremony . . . .

   The next words will be

   A. the sponsor of the event chose
   B. a group was chosen
   C. would be chosen by the sponsor
   D. students from Argentina chose

GO ON TO THE NEXT PAGE

5. I had read his latest book, and after checking on many facts that he cited, decided he was not an author to be trusted.

Rewrite, beginning with

<u>After reading his latest book and checking on many facts that he cited,</u> . . . .

The next words will be

  A. the author's trust
  B. the decision
  C. I decided
  D. trusting the author

6. Dr. Rodriguez believed that his diagnosis was correct, but he doubted that any of the available medication would remedy the condition.

Rewrite, beginning with

<u>Although doubting that any of the available medication would remedy the condition,</u> . . . .

The next words will be

  A. his diagnosis
  B. it would
  C. and Dr. Rodriguez
  D. Dr. Rodriguez

7. My grandparents would be in shock when they learned that they had spent their life savings on worthless shares of a gold mine.

Rewrite, beginning with

<u>To learn they had spent their life savings on worthless shares of a gold mine.</u> . . . .

The next words will be

  A. leaving my grandparents
  B. shock would have left
  C. would leave my grandparents
  D. it would shock

8. The salesperson, being too eager to help the prospective customer, thoughtlessly left the open cash register unattended.

Rewrite, beginning with

<u>The open cash register was thoughtlessly left open.</u> . . . .

The next words will be

  A. by the salesperson, who
  B. , and the salesperson was
  C. eagerly by the salesperson
  D. by the eagerness of the salesperson

9. Weather conditions prevented the scientists from viewing the crater of the volcano at close range.

Rewrite, beginning with

Because of weather conditions, ...

The next words will be

   A.   the crater of the volcano could not be viewed

   B.   scientists could not view the crater of the volcano

   C.   viewing of the crater of the volcano

   D.   to view the crater of the volcano

10. A team of firefighters was sent by the head of operations to check on the status of homes on the other side of the highway.

Rewrite, beginning with

To check on the status of homes on the other side of the highway . . . .

The next words will be

   A.   a team of firefighters was sent

   B.   was sent by the head of operations

   C.   sending a team of firefighters

   D.   the head of operations sent

11. After the performance of the new play, the audience, which had squirmed uncomfortably throughout, burst into applause.

Rewrite, beginning with

Squirming uncomfortably throughout the new play, ...

The next word will be

   A.   a burst of applause

   B.   the audience

   C.   the performance

   D.   it caused the audience

12. A new theater which will provide a space for the acting company is being planned for next year.

Rewrite, beginning with

Planned for next year, ...

   A.   a new theater will provide

   B.   a space for the acting company

   C.   the acting company will be provided

   D.   and to provide space

GO ON TO THE NEXT PAGE

Part B

Directions: In each of the following questions, select the best version of the underlined part of the sentence. Choice A is the same as the underlined portion of the original sentence. If you think the original sentence is best, choose A.

13. Ski resorts in the area drew hundreds of visitors because of the heavy snowfall, <u>and it lasted</u> almost a week.

    A. and it lasted
    B. and the snowfall lasted
    C. which lasted
    D. it lasted

14. Because after a long debate the council members had approved the idea, <u>and they were ready</u> to move on to the next issue.

    A. and they were ready
    B. they were ready
    C. the next issue was ready
    D. therefore they were ready

15. Some of the fans painted their faces, dyed their hair green, and <u>loudly chanting the school's fight song</u> throughout the game.

    A. loudly chanting the school's fight song
    B. then they were loudly chanting the school's fight song
    C. loudly chanted the school's fight song
    D. and throughout the game loudly chanting

16. <u>Viewing the neighborhood from a helicopter,</u> I was amazed by the changes that had occurred since the fire.

    A. Viewing the neighborhood from a helicopter,
    B. As the neighborhood was viewed from a helicopter,
    C. When I was viewing the neighborhood from a helicopter,
    D. To view the neighborhood from a helicopter,

17. The coach recommended <u>that we get plenty of rest, practicing at least three hours a day, and eating</u> a high-carbohydrate breakfast before the meet.

    A. that we get plenty of rest, practicing at least three hours a day, and eating
    B. getting plenty of rest, practicing at least three hours a day, and eat
    C. get plenty of rest, practice at least three hours a day and that we should eat
    D. get plenty of rest, practice at least three hours a day, and eat

18. In his ruling that the state had a right to annex Wilson's property, <u>support was provided by Judge Ryan by citing several precedents</u>.

    A. support was provided by Judge Ryan by citing several precedents
    B. Judge Ryan cited several precedents as support
    C. several precedents, as support, were cited by Judge Ryan
    D. Judge Ryan supported the citing of several precedents

19. Hurricanes are not common occurrences in that part of the country, <u>therefore, people are not</u> adequately prepared to deal with them.

    A.   therefore, people are not
    B.   and therefore people are not
    C.   meaning therefore people are not
    D.   which means that therefore people are not

20. As soon as <u>the party-goers had left the hotel rooms, the maids cleaned them</u> thoroughly.

    A.   the party-goers had left the hotel rooms, the maids cleaned them
    B.   the hotel rooms were left by the party-goers
    C.   the party-goers had left, the maids cleaned them
    D.   the party-goers had left, the maids cleaned the hotel rooms

21. During the summer they spent in Italy, they discovered that the local wines, which were inexpensive, <u>and they surpassed</u> the high-priced ones they were accustomed to drinking.

    A.   and they surpassed
    B.   and were surpassing
    C.   surpassed
    D.   surpassing

22. Suddenly realizing that the price of the car didn't include <u>tax, it caused</u> Procter to rethink his decision to purchase it.

    A.   tax, it caused
    B.   tax caused
    C.   tax, causing
    D.   tax, which caused

23. At the small local movie theater, attendance was lower than the previous year because of <u>higher ticket prices and that people preferred</u> the new cineplex.

    A.   higher ticket prices and that people preferred
    B.   higher ticket prices and people preferred
    C.   higher ticket prices and the preference by people for
    D.   higher ticket prices and people's preference for

24. The policeman chased the suspect for several blocks, <u>during which he repeatedly fired</u> his weapon.

    A.   during which he repeatedly fired
    B.   repeatedly firing his weapon
    C.   the policeman was repeatedly firing
    D.   during the chase repeatedly firing

GO ON TO THE NEXT PAGE

Part C

Directions: Each of the following questions presents a passage with a missing sentence indicated by a series of dashes. Read each passage and the four sentences that follow it. Then choose the sentence that can best be inserted in place of the dashes.

25. Over hundreds of years California has been "invaded" by non-native animal species, some of which can cause problems for native species. - - - - On the other hand, parakeets and parrots, which came from Mexico, Central and South America, India and Africa, and which were set free into the wilds of California, are not considered a threat at this time. Neither is the Virginia opossum, which was probably introduced in California as a game animal.

   A. Animals from other environments provide interest and diversity and often adjust so well that most people think they are native to the state.

   B. The largest frog in North America, the bullfrog, is not native to California but arrived in the state in the late 1800's.

   C. The house sparrow, for example, came west with the railroads, and is bad for native bird species because it takes over their nest sites.

   D. The house mouse, originally from Central Asia, doesn't compete with native species because of its affinity for living near people.

26. In the 1950s, Las Vegas was known as a place you could count on for cheap, hearty buffets, even if the food itself wasn't necessarily first class. Hotels offered bargain buffets at meal times even as the casinos were more than happy to empty your pockets at slot machines and gaming tables. - - - - Food will probably never replace gambling as the city's number one attraction, but "fine dining" is now another drawing card for the desert city.

   A. For some time, however, Las Vegas has been a serious dining city, where some of the best chefs in the country have opened spectacular restaurants.

   B. According to statistics and popular wisdom, visitors have little chance to win a fortune, but hope springs eternal for people who love to gamble.

   C. Floor shows in Las Vegas continue to draw some of the biggest names in show business.

   D. If you can't afford a trip to Paris or Italy or the pyramids, Las Vegas presents an imitation version on a grand scale.

27. - - - -The pika's habitat is in mountain slopes strewn with rocks, but it is being pushed to higher elevations and running out of places to live. Intrusions such as roads close to their habitat and pressure from grazing livestock are partly responsible. Also, pikas, which are very sensitive to high temperatures, may be one of the best early warning systems for detecting global warming in the western United States. Archeologist Donald K. Grayson says the distribution of pikas in the Great Basin has diminished, and 7 of 25 historically described populations appear to have become extinct by the end of the 20th century.

A. The area between the Sierra Nevada mountain range and the Rocky Mountains is referred to as the Great Basin.

B. Human activity and climate change appear to be pushing a small rabbit-like mammal, called a pika, towards extinction.

C. Today, archeologists are among the scientists involved in the study of global warming.

D. The Great Basin pika populations are isolated on separated mountain ranges, and they cannot get to one another.

28. Jane Austen (1775-1817) was at ease in her world. She spent most of her life in the countryside of southern England, a pleasant green landscape where villages, each centered around a church, suggested a feeling of social and family solidarity. - - - - Austen, very different from the conventional idea of literary genius or a tortured soul flailing against the world, produced enduring works that comment with wit and good sense on her social surroundings.

A. Austen herself lived in a lively and affectionate family.

B. The society around Steventon, where Austen lived, had its share of fools and pedants.

C. Nearly half of Jane Austen's grown-up life was after 1800.

D. In Austen's world a clergyman was seen less as a dedicated priest and more as a citizen who represented society in its religious and moral aspects, much as a lawyer represented it in its legal aspects.

GO ON TO THE NEXT PAGE

29. W.E. Burghardt Du Bois' *The Souls of Black Folk,* published in 1903, is recognized as a moving portrait of African-Americans in search of themselves in an alien world and of their often bitter struggle for human rights. One writer describes *The Souls of Black Folks* as "more history-making than historical" because it fixed "that moment in history where the American Negro began to reject the idea of the world's belonging to white people only." - - - -

  A. W.E.B. DuBois, while at Harvard, wrote his dissertation on the suppression of the slave trade, and it was chosen as the first volume of the new Harvard Historical Studies (1896).

  B. DuBois grew up in the period following the Civil War and Reconstruction.

  C. With the book's publication, African-Americans of training and intelligence found a bond in their grievances and a language in which to express them.

  D. Booker T. Washington, who was the most important African-American leader at the time, is the subject of perhaps DuBois' most famous essay.

30. A few early inventions arose simply from the handling of raw materials. For example, pottery probably came about as a result of people in different areas observing the properties of clay, a widespread natural material. More complex inventions, however, such as writing and the wheel were probably the result of borrowing, because these inventions spread more rapidly in the Old World than they could have been invented independently. - - - -

  A. The early Old World wheels have a peculiar design, basically a wooden circle made of three planks.

  B. Door locks, pulleys, and windmills came from a single West Asian source.

  C. One reason that useful inventions spread is that other societies saw or learned of the invention, were receptive to it, and adopted it.

  D. Throughout history, inventions have been of vital importance in man's attempts to deal successfully with the world around him.

31. Chess was invented in India in the 5th century. Through Islamic conquests, the game spread to Europe where an interesting change occurred. Late in the 10th century, during the regency of Empress Adelaide, the chess piece known as the vizier became the queen, and the queen became the only female in the all-male club of chess pieces.- - - - Whereas the queen was at first a piece that took one timid diagonal step at a time on the chessboard, she became the most powerful piece, making the game much faster and more competitive.

   A. Marilyn Yalom, in her book *Birth of the Chess Queen,* sets forth the theory that the change of the chess piece reflects the growth of powerful female European monarchs.

   B. In her book *Birth of the Chess Queen,* Marilyn Yalom presents a lively history of one of the most popular board games.

   C. Marilyn Yalom, in *Birth of the Chess Queen,* explains the origins of each of the pieces in chess.

   D. A vizier is a high executive officer of some Muslim countries, particularly the Ottoman Empire.

32. The Union Conscription Act (1863) provided that all able-bodied men between 20 and 45 could be drafted into military service in the Union Army. If, however, a man could furnish an acceptable substitute or pay the government $300, he could avoid service. To say the law was unpopular is an understatement. It led to nationwide disturbances. Not surprisingly, the riots were especially bloody and violent in New York. - - - -

   A. President Lincoln supported a Democratic commission that investigated the draft in New York City.

   B. The privilege of buying one's way out of service was limited to conscientious objectors in 1864.

   C. Many elements in New York sympathized with the South, and the war had aggravated social and economic grievances.

   D. The Democrat Horatio Seymour was governor of New York at the time of the 1863 draft riots.

GO ON TO THE NEXT PAGE

33. - - - - First born children, for example, are more likely to attend college than children in other positions in a family. A middle child may feel that life is unfair because he or she has neither the rights of the oldest nor the privileges of the youngest. In larger families, however, middle children may be less competitive because parents don't have as much time to give them and so therefore they learn to cooperate to get what they want. The youngest child in a family may feel weak or inferior because every one else is bigger and more capable. At the same time, however, "the baby" often becomes the boss by getting the others to do things for him or her.

A. Generalizations about the effect of birth order, sometimes referred to as ordinal position, can be dangerous.

B. Parents should attempt to see each of their children as a unique individual and avoid making comparisons.

C. The oldest child in a family enjoys the best position for several reasons, among them that he or she, as an only child for a while, enjoys the parents' undivided attention.

D. Researchers have come to some interesting conclusions by studying the effect of birth order on personality and behavior.

34. When I graduated from high school, my parents urged me to enjoy myself during the summer before I was to enter college. It was as if I were the condemned man who deserved a good last meal before his execution. This wasn't because they thought college was a miserable, grueling experience but because they knew (or hoped) that soon enough, I would be pulling all-nighters and spending endless hours at the library. - - - -

A. My parents were proud of my high-school performance and the fact that I'd been accepted at the university.

B. I was perfectly willing to go along with my parents' thinking, of course, because it meant a summer of freedom and good times.

C. My older brother had not only been an outstanding athlete in college but also an honor student.

D. I decided to apply for a summer job with the local newspaper because I planned to make journalism my career some day.

35. After the historic Lewis and Clark expedition, President Thomas Jefferson rewarded both men handsomely with large parcels of land and double pay. - - - - The lives of the two men, however, went in different directions. Lewis went into debt buying land and getting the expedition journals ready for publication. When he sought reimbursement for expense money, Secretary of War William Eustis intimated that he would profit from the funds. Severely depressed, Lewis committed suicide. Clark, on the other hand, became the leading federal official in the west for six presidents, from Jefferson to Van Buren.

   A. Captain Meriwether Lewis was appointed governor of the Territory of Upper Louisiana and Captain William Clark governor of the Missouri Territory.

   B. The expedition journals were sent to Clark after Lewis' death and were presented to the public in 1814, 10 years after the beginning of the epic journey.

   C. Another member of the expedition, Sgt. John Ordway, sold his journal to Lewis and Clark for $300.

   D. Clark's biographer, Landon Y. Jones, says that the presidents Clark served under trusted him to protect American interests in the territory.

36. - - - - Recently scientists identified a defective gene that appears to cause hemochromatosis, or iron overload. Iron overload is fairly easily cured if it is recognized and treated early, but currently it is often misdiagnosed because it mimics more familiar conditions. When not treated in time, iron overload leads to a number of diseases, from diabetes to liver cancer. By identifying the faulty gene through a screening test, physicians will be able to determine patients who carry it and treat them before hemochromatosis worsens.

   A. Physicians today must be well acquainted with gene therapy.

   B. Hemochromastosis, or iron overload, is not understood by most people.

   C. Identification of particular genes can lead to better medicine.

   D. Modern medicine has made remarkable progress.

GO ON TO THE NEXT PAGE

Part D

Directions: Each of the following questions presents a topic and four sentences. Select the sentence that provides the best support for the topic presented.

37. Many people look back to their childhoods as idyllic times when life was filled with pleasure.

    A. Accepting the responsibilities of adulthood is necessary if one wants to be treated as an adult.

    B. Psychologists say that the first years of a child's life are instrumental in his or her adjustment in later life.

    C. Children often understand more than adults think they do.

    D. Collecting dolls, toy cars, or stuffed animals can be a way of trying to recapture the past.

38. The violent eruption of Mt. St. Helen's volcano in May of 1980 had several immediate effects.

    A. Mt. St. Helen's peak was reduced from 9,677 feet to 8,325 feet.

    B. In 1986, the volcano fell silent, and then in 2004, low-level earthquakes began.

    C. Weather conditions often prevent aerial observation of the volcanic crater at Mt. St. Helen.

    D. About one-tenth of the world's volcanoes are in the United States.

39. According to many political scientists and commentators, elections are often influenced by factors that have little to do with major issues.

    A. Polls monitor closely the effect of political debates.

    B. To an undecided voter, someone who always supports one party may seem to be a fanatic.

    C. One poll found that only 30 percent of voters named an issue when they explained why they voted as they did.

    D. The most widely known fact about George H.W. Bush in the 1992 election, according to polls, was that he hated broccoli.

40. Being raised by a single parent was, for me, not without benefits.

    A. Evening meals were often prepared (and eaten) on the run, since my mother's working hours constantly varied.

    B. Friends weren't allowed to visit my house when my mother wasn't home.

    C. Very early I learned how to cook, clean, do laundry, and shop wisely.

    D. Our apartment was big enough for my mother and me.

41. When people oppose legislation designed to protect the environment, they set forth what appear to be legitimate arguments.

    A. Evidence supporting the fact that our earth is warming is overwhelming, according to experts.

    B. Limiting oil exploration and drilling in the United States may increase our dependence on other countries, according to some commentators.

    C. Environmentalists have stepped up their efforts in recent years, but those efforts have sometimes failed.

    D. Efforts to control air pollution have produced promising results, but the problem is ongoing, particularly in heavily urban areas.

42. American students usually study European languages in public schools, but there are signs that this could change.

    A. China is rapidly emerging as a global superpower in this century.

    B. Experts agree that the younger a child is, the easier it is to introduce him to a second language.

    C. Education officials should try for more teacher exchanges with other countries.

    D. Some urban school districts have launched programs in Mandarin Chinese.

43. Some modern inventions actually have ancient origins.

    A. Otis invented the modern elevator and successfully demonstrated it in 1854, while the first escalator dates from the 1890's.

    B. Tracing inventions to their sources is a fascinating, if sometimes frustrating, pursuit.

    C. The idea of a parking meter, for example, goes back to an ancient Greek scientist who built a machine that delivered a cupful of holy water on inserting a coin.

    D. Many inventions have made life easier, but some, such as the telescope, have led to astounding discoveries about the universe.

44. The Public Broadcasting System (PBS) was created with specific goals and directives.

    A. Some critics have described network television as a "vast wasteland."

    B. Public television should, in the words of the 1967 Public Broadcasting Act, "have instructional, educational, and cultural purposes" and take "creative risks."

    C. In recent years, PBS has been described by some opponents as serving a small, elite group at the expense of all taxpayers.

    D. Local public television stations pay dues to the Corporation for Public Broadcasting in return for services and broadcasting rights.

45. The process of finding a job is still daunting for me, even though I have done it several times.

    A. Being interviewed by a prospective employer sends chills down my spine.

    B. Opportunities are listed on various Internet sites, something not available to my grandparents.

    C. I research the company where I'm applying for a job before I prepare a resume.

    D. My most successful interviews are those in which I'm able to let my personality show through.

IF YOU FINISH BEFORE TIME IS CALLED, CHECK YOUR WORK ON THIS SECTION ONLY. DO NOT WORK ON ANY OTHER SECTION IN THE TEST.

Answer Key: Sample Essay and Evaluation in Explanation Section

Reading Skills

Type 1: Short Reading Passages (Part A)

1. C
2. A
3. A
4. B
5. C
6. A
7. B
8. C

9. B
10. C
11. A
12. C
13. D
14. C
15. A

Type II: Vocabulary in Context (Part B)

16. C
17. A
18. C
19. D
20. A
21. D
22. B
23. C

24. A
25. C
26. B
27. D
28. A
29. C
30. D

Type III: Sentence Relationships (Part C)

31. A
32. C
33. D
34. B
35. A
36. D
37. C
38. A

39. B
40. A
41. B
42. C
43. D
44. B
45. A

Composing Skills

Type I: Construction Shift (Part A)

1. B		**7.** C	
2. C		**8.** A	
3. D		**9.** B	
4. A		**10.** D	
5. C		**11.** C	
6. D		**12.** A	

Type II: Sentence Correction (Part B)

13. C		**19.** B	
14. B		**20.** D	
15. C		**21.** C	
16. A		**22.** B	
17. D		**23.** D	
18. B		**24.** B	

Type III: Missing Sentence (Part C)

25. C		**31.** A	
26. A		**32.** C	
27. B		**33.** D	
28. A		**34.** B	
29. C		**35.** A	
30. C		**36.** C	

Type IV: Supporting Sentence (Part D)

37. D		**42.** D	
38. A		**43.** C	
39. C		**44.** B	
40. C		**45.** A	
41. B			

Analyzing Your Test Results

Use the following charts to carefully analyze your results and spot your strengths and weaknesses. Complete the process of analyzing each subject area and each individual question for the Practice Test. Examine your results for trends in types of error (repeated errors) or poor results in specific subject areas. This re-examination and analysis is of tremendous importance for effective test preparation.

The Essay

See the discussion of essay scoring beginning on page 179 to evaluate your essays. Have someone knowledgeable in reading instruction read and evaluate your responses using the essay scoring guide on page 180.

Practice Test Analysis Sheet: Reading Skills

Reading Skills				
	Possible	Completed	Right	Wrong
Reading Passages	15			
Vocabulary in Context	15			
Sentence Relationships	15			
Total:	45			

Analysis/Tally Sheet for Multiple-Choice Questions

One of the most important parts of test preparation is analyzing *why* you missed a question so that you can reduce the number of mistakes. Now that you've taken the Practice Test and corrected your answers, carefully tally your multiple-choice mistakes by marking in the proper column.

Reasons for Mistakes				
	Total Missed	Simple Mistake	Misread Problem	Lack of Knowledge
Reading Passages				
Vocabulary in Context				
Sentence Relationships				
Total:				

Practice Test Analysis Sheet: Composing Skills

Composing Skills				
	Possible	*Completed*	*Right*	*Wrong*
Construction Shift	12			
Sentence Correction	12			
Missing Sentence	12			
Supporting Sentence	9			
Total:	45			

Analysis/Tally Sheet for Multiple-Choice Questions

One of the most important parts of test preparation is analyzing *why* you missed a question so that you can reduce the number of mistakes. Now that you've taken the Practice Test and corrected your answers, carefully tally your multiple-choice mistakes by marking in the proper column.

Reasons for Mistakes				
	Total Missed	*Simple Mistake*	*Misread Problem*	*Lack of Knowledge*
Construction Shift				
Sentence Correction				
Missing Sentence				
Supporting Sentence				
Total:				

Explanation of Answers

Sample Student Essay

Colin Magnus calls into question whether having information is always good for us and whether too much of it may actually be counterproductive. The question is if information is all it's cracked up to be. And an extension of that question is this: Is a lack of information, that is quiet, sometimes to be preferred? On the face of it, the proposal that less information is better seems absurd, but Mr. Magnus has a point. When we are overloaded with input sometimes we tune it out and don't remember any of it— we "crash" like an overloaded computer memory chip.

Information can, of course, be good, and often essential. We must have correct information to function day to day. We must know how to cook a meal, and write a letter, and choose something to wear that's right for the weather, and get from here to there and not get lost. We must have enough information to do our jobs to earn enough money to live. Not many of us would choose to give up our computers these days or our iPods or our TVs and DVDs and cell phones. The very idea would probably make most of us uncomfortable. But . . . maybe we should learn to turn them off. Maybe there's a time when the "noise" Magnus speaks of gets so overwhelming that it gets in the way of thought.

In the connected world of TV news and instant reporting on everything that's happening and the constant playing of the same songs on the radio and the showing of the same movies all over the country at the same time, we all have exactly the same experiences and receive the same input day to day. This sameness can lead to a loss of individuality and a lack of independent thinking. For example, if in an election one station comes out with an announcement of the winner, all the others tend to get right in line and say that's the winner too, even if nobody actually knows and even if the first station was wrong and didn't have the facts to back it up. If two or three people at school say something is true about somebody else, we tend to think it automatically is. Just because we hear something that's supposedly "information," that doesn't mean it's true. But because we hear things over and over and over, somehow we assume that they are true. It's how urban legends get started. There's an old saying, "Don't believe everything you read in the paper." Now it might be, "Don't believe everything you see on the Internet."

I think everyone has had the experience of saying something like "there's so much noise in here I can't think" or at least wanting to say "don't tell me any more about it—I'm trying to absorb what you told me already." Can we "know" too much? Probably not, if it's true knowledge. But can we hear and see too much, every hour of every day? Yes, we can. Thoreau found a life of quiet reflection at Walden Pond of great value. We might find that at least an hour or two a day without the electronic "noise" leads to our being able to use the essential information to our advantage and learning to trust our own quiet thought processes.

Analysis of the Student Essay

This writer in the first sentence demonstrates a clear understanding of the topic. The writer also quickly sees the problem raised by Magnus, that of the possibility of too much information. The underlying question isn't whether information itself is bad but rather if too much of it can be overwhelming.

The essay is well organized. It first examines what Magnus is saying and takes a stand, suggesting that while the statements at first might seem "absurd," they may have some merit. The essay goes on to investigate what that merit might be and gives good examples of why some information is essential. The writer has good control of language and usage, using conversational style, as in "all it's cracked up to be" and interesting phrasing as in "crash like an overloaded computer memory chip." The essay also uses excellent specific references to such things as DVDs and the Internet.

The essay may get somewhat off track in the third paragraph, with the emphasis on whether information is true or not and the repetition concerning this point, but the general idea is well enough connected to the thesis that the overload of information can be a bad thing that it isn't distracting from the essay's thesis as a whole.

The fourth paragraph nicely brings the essay to a close, citing personal experiences and using the appropriate reference to the quiet of Thoreau's Walden Pond.

Reading Skills

Type I: Short Reading Passages (Part A)

1. **C.** The context does not suggest that egregious errors are "lively and amusing" (A). Choices B and D are too specific; the errors described in the passage are bad, but nothing indicates they are "provocative" or "confrontational."

2. **A.** The author specifically states that the thesaurus is helpful, not "useless" (B), and nothing is said to indicate it is "overly praised" or "inadequately researched" (C, D). The point that the author does make is that Roget's Thesaurus, because of its organization, is not as easy to use as a modern A-Z thesaurus.

3. **A.** After stating that a modern thesaurus is easier to use than Roget's, the author of the passage points out that greater convenience does not eliminate a basic problem with any thesaurus: users choosing inappropriate synonyms.

4. **B.** In stating that some teachers think Roget might have created a "monster," the author of the passage is using figurative, rather than literal, language. None of the other sentences (A, C, and D) make use of a metaphor.

5. **C.** Mentioning "honeymoons" in a passage that focuses on a mummy points out the oddness of the mummy's location. Choices A and B are weak. If the author were trying to locate the site of the museum, he/she would perhaps say "upstate New York," and if he/she were pointing out the attractions of Niagara Falls, "honeymoon spot" would certainly not be the only (or main) one. Choice D is simply wrong; the author doesn't "poke fun" at anyone.

6. **A.** The passage does illustrate the popularity of Egyptian culture (C), but this is not the author's primary purpose. Also, the author doesn't touch on the "dangers" of tomb raiding (B), nor does he/she show proof that the mummy is Rameses I (D). The author's intention is to relate an interesting historical anecdote.

7. **B.** That Lincoln, Grant, and P.T. Barnum visited the collection implies the popularity of mummies. The other choices aren't implied in the passage. Dr. James Douglas "acquired" the mummy for the museum, but there is no suggestion that he actually looted the tomb (A). The author does not imply that the mummy may not be Rameses I (C) but in fact accepts the idea that he is. See the last sentence. Nothing suggests that Cairo "fought vigorously" for the mummy's return (D).

8. **C.** It is a primary definition of "murky," and of the choices offered, is the one that makes the best sense in context. Choice B is too strong a word, and the examples of "looting, illegal purchase, and neglect" do not fit well with "surprisingly lucky" or "not researched" (A, D).

9. **B.** The presentation of the information is factual. The final sentence, though it could suggest an irony (C), does not reflect the tone of the passage as a whole. The tone is neither "reverent" nor "sentimental" (A, D).

10. **C.** Whereas people can now get an excellent glimpse of pre-Columbian South America, accessibility has brought with it efforts to turn Machu Picchu into a tourist attraction. It has also has led to damage of one of the city's treasures. Choice B is irrelevant, and Choice A is not touched upon in the passage. Although the trip to Machu Picchu is both difficult and rewarding (D), this is not as good an example of what is meant by "mixed blessing."

11. **A.** The author does not expect an answer to this question. Instead, it is a comment on what has happened to the Incan "retreat." None of the other choices describes accurately the last sentence of the passage.

12. **C.** Choices A and D may seem to be good answers, but it isn't known whether "most people" believe in the city nor is it clear that no one will ever find it. "Fabled" suggests that it is widely believed and talked about but it isn't clear whether such a "lost city" actually exists.

13. **D.** The author states the point of the passage in the first sentence. He/She does not actually describe the system (A), and although he/she does make a comparison, the comparison is not the main purpose. One thing the author does not do in the passage is explain the effect of granting too many patents (C).

14. **C.** According to the theory, an inventor is motivated to create if he/she can be the sole proprietor of the idea. That ownership translates into money. Patents provide the assurance that the inventor will be rewarded. The other choices are simply not relevant to an inventor's motivation.

15. **A.** The author does make comparisons, suggest that understaffing is one reason so many patents are granted, and express his opinion that too many patents are granted (B, C, and D). The only thing that he does not do is explain why issuing so many patents is a bad idea.

Type II: Vocabulary in Context (Part B)

16. C. The words "innocent" and "sweet" rule out Choice B. Choices A and D are also inappropriate in a sentence where the emphasis is on sweetness and innocence.

17. A. It is unlikely that choices B and D remarks would be "boring," and Choice C is less likely than Choice A, which means dull, flat.

18. C. One of its meanings is not physically active, which fits the context here. Choice B might seem a good answer. "Languid" means drooping or flagging as if from exhaustion, but its connotations suggest listlessness or a sluggish disposition.

19. D. It means beyond realism, strange, or dreamlike. (Surrealism is in fact a term given to an artistic movement in which the works use fantastic or dreamlike images.) Neither choices A nor C fits the context at all. Choice B, literally meaning rotten, can figuratively mean morally corrupt or totally objectionable, but these meanings also don't fit the context ("wild dream") well.

20. A. Choices B, C, and D don't describe "clinging" to a belief. "Tenaciously" in this context means persistently.

21. D. "The atmosphere of the city" is likely to be cosmopolitan, which means worldly, sophisticated, not provincial. Although one might like this aspect of the city, one is unlikely to like (or miss) the congestion (B). Choice A doesn't make much sense here; literate means able to read or widely read, but these are not necessarily associated with "the city." Choice C refers to a deteriorating area that has been renewed or rebuilt for middle- and upper-class tenants.

22. B. Choice C means something opposite to the context, and Choice D is irrelevant. Choice A, which means pleasant or amiable, is more appropriate in describing an individual than a group. Choice B stresses the ability to work harmoniously with a group.

23. C. Retract describes a publication's taking back a story after it has been released. Choice A, while possible, is not as appropriate; the actor would certainly want more than a "repositioning" of the story. Choice B can mean to deny the existence or truth of something, but it is not accurate in this context. Choice D doesn't make sense here.

24. A. To impede is to interfere with the progress of something. Choice C's meaning is opposite to the idea in the sentence. Choice D is simply too strong; it suggests a more forceful move. Choice B makes little sense in this context.

25. C. "Stringent" means very strict, rigid and is often used in reference to rules and regulations. The second-best answer would be Choice A, which means strong or powerful, but it is not as precise a word in this context. Choices B and D are irrelevant.

26. B. The account moved Joanne almost to tears, and Choice B means deeply moving. While Choice A might deeply affect a reader, it's unlikely it would move her to tears. A realistic account (D) might also move a reader, but it is less precise here than Choice B. Choice C does not fit the context well.

27. D. In this situation (context), asking her father for her hand would seem archaic to Pamela, that is, out-of-date, surviving from an earlier period. Choice B might seem a good answer, but it is too strong. Choices A and C don't fit the context; "opportune" means suitable or convenient for a particular occurrence and "unwieldy" means not easily handled or managed.

28. A. Travails are tasks, usually difficult ones. This word fits the particular context (with the mention of the handsome stranger and the princess) better than the more mundane "tasks." Choice C might seem a good choice, since answering riddles often wins heroes the maiden in fairy tales, but riddles do not involve "every aspect of . . . character and strength."

29. C. This question is related to a spelling problem. Whereas Choice C means to come before, Choice A means to move ahead, continue. These two words are often confused. Choice D means to rule out in advance and Choice B to catch up with, neither of which works in context.

30. D. It means frank, honest, unreserved. The sentence states that his friends admire Carlos, which would likely rule out Choice A. Choice B is a possibility, but in this context humility would be less admirable than candor. Choice C (logic) doesn't describe Carlos's statement that the experiment was flawed.

Type III: Sentence Relationships (Part C)

31. A. The second sentence is an example of a widening pay gap, not an exception to it. Choice C is not a good answer because the second sentence, although it specifically deals with women "of varied mathematical skills," doesn't introduce a new idea; it focuses on the widening pay gap. No conclusion (B) is drawn regarding the widening pay gap.

32. C. A different point of view that regulation of the Internet is not a good idea is suggested in the second sentence. It questions, but does not refute (D), the first statement, and it is not introducing an exception (B) but an entirely different point of view. No comparison (A) is made.

33. D. The second sentence doesn't support or offer an illustration of Hamlet's rejection (B, A) but states an effect. What is the effect of Hamlet's rejection of Ophelia? She kills herself.

34. B. Although the second sentence doesn't begin "The reason is . . . .," the implication is clear that the increased consumption of wood is at least one cause of depleted old-growth forests. At first glance Choice A may seem correct, but note that the increased wood consumption is not an example of how the United States is losing old-growth forests but one reason for the loss.

35. A. Clearly, the reception to the second half of the play is being contrasted to the reception to the first half. None of the other answers is relevant. The negative reaction to the second half of the play is certainly not an illustration (B) or a consequence (D) of the positive reaction to the first half, nor does it refute (C) it.

36. D. Perhaps there are many reasons the writer had difficulty making friends, but the second sentence directly states one of those reasons. It doesn't provide evidence (C) that he/she had difficulties, nor does it draw a parallel (A). A sentence drawing a parallel might be "My older brother had also been a 'loner' when he was in grade school."

37. C. By invalidating Lincoln's suspension of habeas corpus, the Court chose the rule of law rather than the rule of an individual, which supports the statement in the first sentence. The suspension is neither a reason nor a cause (A, B). Nothing is compared in the second sentence.

38. A. Does the second sentence give supporting evidence (C)? No, it simply emphasizes the point in the first sentence, without citing any particular work of science fiction as evidence. It underlines (doesn't provide an exception to) the point of the first sentence (B), and it draws no conclusions (D).

39. B. Two conditions of the family are compared: 10 years ago and today. (Those words are a good clue that a comparison is being made.) Nothing in the second sentence suggests that the family's situation today is a consequence of what happened 10 years ago (C), nor does the second sentence support the first (D) or draw a conclusion about the change (A).

40. A. The word "dispute" is a clue that the second sentence will provide a viewpoint different from the generalization in the first sentence. Choice B might seem a possible answer. But the Rockford students aren't part of a comparison; rather, they question the assumption that is made in the first sentence.

41. B. The second sentence enumerates some of the classes being offered and refers to the low fees. Although the sentence does compare the fees to those of private lessons, its primary purpose is to provide examples, not to compare (C).

42. C. Why are the families wandering aimlessly in the streets? As a consequence of the explosion. Sentence 1, not sentence 2, states the cause (B). The second sentence does more than emphasize the statement in the first (D), and the wandering families are a result, not an example (A).

43. D. Mr. Martin is definitely an exception to the enthusiastic "everyone" of the first sentence. He certainly doesn't emphasize the enthusiasm (A), nor is he an example or consequence of it (B, C).

44. B. There may be an unspoken assumption that because of the changes in the landscape, animals and plants will have disappeared. But the first sentence, not the second, refutes that possible assumption (D). The second sentence then supports the statement by providing specific examples of the diverse life still present.

45. A. The first sentence begins "Some people believe. . . ." The second sentence questions that assumption: "It is more likely that. . . ." This is not a comparison (B) of ideas but a questioning of an idea. The view in the second sentence doesn't emphasize the view presented in the first (D), nor does it provide an example (C); it provides an entirely different view.

Composing Skills

Type I: Construction Shift (Part A)

1. **B.** The sentence begins with a participial phrase and therefore must be followed by the subject of the phrase: "hikers . . . having gathered." Choices A and C indicate that the "warnings," not the hikers, gathered at the foot of the mountain. This error is called a dangling participle. Choice D is incorrect because in this version the pronoun "they" would have no antecedent (word for which it stands).

2. **C.** It directly states what the pilot predicted. Choice A isn't the prediction, and choices B and D, though they aren't grammatically incorrect, are unnecessarily wordy.

3. **D.** It provides the antecedent for "they," and is the only answer that is in the active rather than passive voice. In most cases, the active voice is more efficient than the passive voice: "Some committee members decided" rather than "It was decided by some committee members."

4. **A.** Choices B and C are both in the passive voice, and Choice D changes the meaning; it is not the students from Argentina who are doing the choosing.

5. **C.** It is the only answer that avoids the dangling participle. "I" must follow the clause containing "reading" and "checking."

6. **D.** Don't be misled by the length of the opening clause. Because it contains the participle "doubting," the subject, "Dr. Rodriguez," must open the next clause. Choice A would indicate that the "diagnosis" was doing the doubting. Choice B also creates a dangling participle, and Choice C creates a sentence fragment.

7. **C.** In this version of the sentence, "To learn they had spent. . . ." acts as the subject. It should be followed by the predicate (verb): "would leave. . . ." Choice A would create a fragment, and Choice D includes an unnecessary "it."

8. **A.** In this case, the rewritten version calls for the passive voice. Using a subordinate clause (beginning with "who") is more effective than using an independent clause (beginning with "and," Choice B). Choice C makes no sense, and Choice D is awkward and wordy.

9. **B.** Here, the active voice is more direct and efficient than the passive voice in Choice A, the wordiness that would be caused by Choice C ("viewing of the crater of the volcano could not be done by the scientists"), or the awkwardness of Choice D ("to view the crater of the volcano would not be possible by the scientists").

10. **D.** The infinitive phrase "To check on. . . . ." acts as an adverb explaining why the head of operations sent the firefighters. This version uses the active voice, which is better than Choice A or Choice B, neither of which is grammatically incorrect. But once again, choose the active voice whenever possible.

11. **C.** The audience is doing the squirming, and therefore "the audience" must follow the participial phrase. Neither "a burst of applause" (A) nor "the performance" (D) is squirming.

12. **A.** The phrase "planned for next year" should be followed immediately by the word(s) it describes: "a new theater." Choice C is a case of a misplaced modifier: the acting company is not planned for next year. Choices B and D would each lead to a long, awkward sentence.

Type II: Sentence Correction (Part B)

13. C. The original version consists of two independent clauses. Changing the second to a subordinate clause is better. Choice B makes no improvement (except to specify the "it"), and Choice D creates a run-on sentence (comma splice).

14. B. The original sentence is a fragment because the first clause can't stand alone ("Because after a long debate. . . ."), and the second clause does not solve the problem. Choice D presents the same problem, and Choice C would create an awkward, wordy sentence.

15. C. Similar elements in a sentence should be parallel in structure: painted, dyed, chanted. All the other answers include a nonparallel element: painted, dyed, chanting.

16. A. The original sentence is correct (the participial phrase is followed by its subject) and is the most efficient of the choices. Choices B and C are both wordy, and Choice D isn't clear.

17. D. Similar elements are parallel in structure: get, practice, eat. This is not the case in the other choices.

18. B. Choice B changes the sentence by using the active form of the verb ("cite"). This eliminates wordiness and is less awkward than Choice C. Choice D changes the meaning. Judge Ryan isn't supporting the citing of precedents but supporting his ruling by citing precedents.

19. B. The original sentence is a run-on (comma splice). "Therefore" begins an independent, not a dependent, clause. Choices C and D are wordy. In this sentence, two independent clauses are appropriate and the most efficient expression of the idea.

20. D. The problem in this sentence is unclear pronoun reference. In the original sentence, the "them" could refer to either the party-goers or the hotel rooms. It is much better to clear up any possible (if unlikely) confusion by using the structure of Choice D.

21. C. The original sentence is a fragment because "wines" has no subject. Choice C is the only choice that solves the problem.

22. B. "Suddenly realizing that the price . . ." acts as a noun and the subject of the sentence, and therefore, the pronoun "it" should be deleted. Choices C and D create fragments.

23. D. Parallel elements should be grammatically parallel: prices and preference. Choices A and B are not parallel, and Choice C is wordy.

24. B. The pronoun reference for "he" in the second clause is unclear. Who is repeatedly firing his weapon, the policeman or the suspect? Choice B eliminates the pronoun and makes it clear that the policeman was firing. Choice C does eliminate the pronoun but creates a run-on sentence. Choice D is wordy.

Type III: Missing Sentence (Part C)

25. C. This sentence is the only one that concerns an invading animal that has caused a problem for native species. Note that the following sentence begins with "on the other hand," which is a clue that the missing sentence will use an example of a non-native species that causes a problem. Choices B and D are about non-native animals, but Choice B doesn't address the competition with native species and Choice D specifically says the mouse doesn't compete. Choice A, which could be a topic sentence for a different paragraph, is too general and doesn't follow from the first sentence of this paragraph

26. A. The word "however" is a clue. The missing sentence should deal with dining both because of the topic sentence and the last sentence. Choices B, C, and D deal with other subjects.

27. B. Choice B introduces the pika as well as the subject of the paragraph, which is the effect of human activity and climate change. While Choice D is about the pika, it does not touch upon the effects of activity and climate. Choice A is a peripheral point, not a topic sentence, and Choice C, while it could be a topic sentence if the paragraph were about global warming, doesn't belong here.

28. A. The topic sentence states that Austen was "at ease in her world," and the second sentence deals with feelings of "social and family solidarity." A statement about Austen's family, therefore, is a good fit. Choice B, while true, goes in a different direction ("fools and pedants"). Choices C and D do not logically follow the second sentence.

29. C. Choice C is the most appropriate closing statement because it deals with the effect of DuBois' book. Choices A, B, and D, while they may be good details to use in a paragraph about DuBois, are not about his book.

30. C. Choice C provides a reason for the spread of inventions. Choices A and B both deal with particular inventions, not with the issue of "borrowed" inventions. Choice D is a general statement that doesn't belong in this paragraph.

31. A. Choice A presents a theory to explain why the vizier became the queen, as well as providing the author and title of the book providing the information. Choices B and C do provide those, but they don't deal with the specific role of the queen. Choice C would seem to be good, but notice the final sentence of the paragraph. Choice D is a minor detail.

32. C. Choice C explains why the riots were especially bloody in New York. Choice A deals with the results of the riots in New York, but it doesn't provide an explanation for them. Choices B and D are details that don't follow the previous sentence smoothly.

33. D. While Choice D isn't a particularly effect topic sentence, it does introduce the subject of findings about birth order. Choices A and B may be true, but they are not what the paragraph is about. Choice C is a detail rather than a topic sentence.

34. B. Choice B fits the light tone of the paragraph and effectively follows the preceding sentence. Choices A and D don't fit as well, in either content or tone. Choice C is an irrelevant sentence here.

35. A. Choice A is a detail that concerns the rewards given to both men—and it precedes the main point of the paragraph, which is to contrast the men's fates. None of the other choices fits in this position.

36. C. Choice C serves as a good topic sentence for the example of how important identification of the hemochromatosis gene has been. Choice A may seem correct at first, but the paragraph is about identifying genes, not gene therapy. Choice D is too broad and not as good as Choice C. Choice B makes a point about the disease, but it does not address the importance of gene identification.

Type IV: Supporting Sentence (Part D)

37. D. Choice D provides support for the idea that people are nostalgic about childhood. The other choices don't provide support; they introduce different ideas.

38. A. Note that the topic says "immediate effects." Choice B concerns earthquakes that occurred long after the eruption. Choices C and D don't concern effects of the eruption at all.

39. C. Choice D might appear to be correct because it refers to a trivial fact that was widely known. But notice that it doesn't suggest that George Bush's dislike of broccoli affected people's votes. The only choice that deals with minor factors influencing elections is Choice C. Choices A and B are irrelevant to the topic.

40. C. The only sentence that cites a benefit is Choice C, although the other choices do deal with details about being raised by a single parent. "Not without benefits" is the clue here.

41. B. Choice B sets forth "what appears to be" a legitimate argument against environmental legislation: dependence on other countries for oil. The other choices, while dealing with environmental issues, do not describe arguments used by those who oppose legislation.

42. D. Choice D is a specific example of a sign of change. While Choice A may provide a reason behind the change, it is not an example of an actual modification in foreign language teaching in public schools. Choices B and C are irrelevant to the topic sentence.

43. C. Notice the phrase "for example." That is a good clue here. The parking meter is a specific example of an invention going back to ancient times. Choice A might seem possible, but the 19th century can't truly be designated as "ancient." Choices B and D don't support the topic.

44. B. The topic specifically mentions "specific goals and directives," and that is what Choice B provides. The other choices do not deal with PBS goals but with extraneous issues.

45. A. The topic sentence includes the term "daunting." Choice A clearly supports the point that finding a job is daunting because interviews send chills down the writer's spine. Choices C and D may cover ways in which the writer handles his or her discomfort, but they don't support the topic statement. Choice B is simply off the subject.

PART VI

FINAL PREPARATION

The Final Touches

1. Make sure that you are familiar with the areas covered on the ELM and EPT.

2. Spend the last week of preparation on a general review of the areas covered with emphasis on strengthening your weak areas.

3. Don't cram the night before the exam. It is a waste of time!

4. Start off crisply, working the questions you know first, then going back and trying to answer the others.

5. Try to eliminate one or more choices before you guess, but make sure that you fill in all the answers. There is no penalty for guessing!

6. Underline key words in the questions. Write out important information and make notations. Take advantage of being permitted to write in the test booklet.

7. Make sure that you answer what is being asked.

8. Use an elimination strategy. Cross out incorrect choices immediately: This can keep you from reconsidering a choice that you have already eliminated.

9. Don't get stuck on any one question. They are all of equal value.

10. The key to getting a good score on the ELM and EPT is reviewing properly and practicing. Get the questions right that you can and should get right. A careful review of each part in this book will help you focus during the final week before each exam.